THE GLP-1 REVOLUTION

THE SCIENCE, MY JOURNEY, AND THE TRUTH ABOUT THESE WEIGHT LOSS DRUGS

AVERY CARTER

2025

Legal Disclaimer

This book is for **informational and educational purposes only**. It is not intended to provide **medical advice, diagnosis, or treatment**. The information contained within is based on research, personal experiences, and publicly available data but should **not** be considered a substitute for professional medical guidance.

Readers should **consult their physician or a qualified healthcare provider** before making any changes to their healthcare, including the use of any medications discussed in this book. The author and publisher assume **no responsibility** for any adverse effects, health outcomes, or decisions made based on the information presented.

Additionally, any names, personal stories, or experiences shared in this book have been **altered, fictionalized, or presented in a way that protects individual privacy**. Any resemblance to actual persons, living or deceased, is purely **coincidental**.

The information in this edition has been **researched and verified up to March 2025**. While every effort has been made to ensure accuracy, medical science and pharmaceutical developments continue to evolve. **Readers are encouraged to verify any medical information with up-to-date sources or consult a healthcare professional.**

The author and publisher make no warranties about the completeness, accuracy, or reliability of the content and expressly disclaim any liability for errors or omissions.

By reading this book, you acknowledge that you assume full responsibility for your health decisions and understand that the author and publisher are **not liable** for any outcomes resulting from the application of the information provided.

QUESTIONS ANSWERED IN THIS BOOK

1. Are weight loss drugs safe long-term, and what are the biggest health risks?
2. How do these medications work, and who is an ideal candidate?
3. What are the most popular weight loss drugs today, and how do they compare?
4. What are the most common side effects, and how can they be managed?
5. Can weight loss drugs lead to sustainable results, or does the weight return after stopping?
6. How do hormones, psychology, and the food industry contribute to weight gain—and how can they be addressed?
7. What role does Big Pharma play in the weight loss industry, and how does it shape public perception?
8. How can weight loss medications be effectively combined with lifestyle changes for lasting success?
9. Are there alternative or holistic approaches to weight loss that work as well as medication?
10. How can individuals take a balanced, informed approach to weight management without falling for hype or misinformation?
11. Bonus article on the trend of micro-dosing GLP-1 drugs.

TABLE OF CONTENTS

INTRODUCTION

Standing in my doctor's office in early 2024, I faced a decision that would transform not just my health but my entire understanding of modern medicine's approach to weight management. After decades of struggling with conventional weight loss methods, I was considering one of the new GLP-1 agonist medications. Like millions of Americans, I had watched these drugs dominate headlines, transform celebrities, and spark intense debates about the future of weight management. But as I learned through my journey, the story of weight loss medication is far more complex – and far more important – than any headline can capture.

The landscape of weight management has undergone a revolutionary transformation. We've moved from the dangerous amphetamine-based pills of the past to sophisticated medications that work with our body's natural systems. This evolution represents more than just medical progress; it reflects a fundamental shift in how we understand obesity, metabolism, and the intricate relationship between our bodies and the food we eat.

As someone who has experienced both the triumphs and challenges of modern weight loss medication, I understand the pressing questions that come with considering these treatments. How safe are these drugs? What happens when you stop taking them? Can they truly offer a lasting solution? These questions deserve thorough, honest answers grounded in both science and real-world experience.

This book emerges from a deep dive into the science, safety, and societal impact of modern weight management medications. Through extensive research and personal experience, I've worked to create a comprehensive guide that goes beyond the basics, examining not just how these medications work but how they fit into the broader context of health, wellness, and our relationship with food.

We'll explore the fascinating science behind how these medications interact with our bodies, the real-world experiences of those who have used them, and the complex interplay between pharmaceutical intervention and lifestyle changes. We'll tackle challenging questions about the role of the pharmaceutical industry and the accessibility of these treatments. Most importantly, we'll explore how these medications fit into a broader approach to health and wellness that acknowledges both the complexity of weight management and the dignity of personal choice.

At its heart, the story of weight loss medication is a human story. It's about people seeking solutions, healthcare providers adapting to new tools, and society grappling with changing perspectives on weight and health. Whether you're considering weight loss medication for yourself, supporting someone who is, or simply seeking to understand this medical revolution, this book aims to provide the knowledge and insights needed to navigate these decisions with confidence.

The weight loss drug revolution is not just about new medications – it's about a fundamental shift in how we approach weight management and health. As we embark on this exploration together, my goal is to provide you with the tools, understanding, and perspective needed to make informed decisions about your health journey. Whether these medications become part of your path or not, understanding their role in modern medicine is crucial for anyone interested in health and wellness in the 21st century.

1

THE EVOLUTION OF WEIGHT LOSS MEDICINE: FROM DIET PILLS TO GLP-1 AGONISTS

The journey of weight loss medicine mirrors humanity's evolving understanding of obesity itself - from a simple matter of willpower to a complex medical condition requiring sophisticated intervention. One of my close friends discovered, in her medical file from 1995, a yellowed prescription for phentermine, a drug similar to an amphetamine that serves as an appetite suppressant. She knew I was researching and brought it up one day over coffee, horrified that it had been a solution for her at one time. It served as a great reminder of how far we've come from the days when diet pills were our only pharmaceutical option for weight management. This transformation in our understanding reflects a broader shift in medical science, moving away from quick-fix solutions toward more sophisticated, targeted approaches that acknowledge obesity as a complex medical condition requiring comprehensive treatment.

Sarah Martinez's discovery in her aunt's attic perfectly illustrates this evolution. As she sorted through old family photographs and documents, she found a small tin box containing dozens of diet pill bottles and handwritten weight loss journals spanning from the 1960s through the 1990s. Each bottle told a story - from the dangerous rainbow pills of the '60s to the fen-phen combinations of the '90s. Her grandmother's journals revealed the emotional rollercoaster these medications created: initial excitement over rapid weight loss, followed by crushing disappointment of regain, and sometimes frightening side effects. Yet the final entry from 2022 painted a different picture - one of success with a GLP-1 agonist medication under proper medical supervision, reflecting not just weight loss achievement but a transformed relationship with food and body awareness.

This journey from dangerous quick fixes to science-based solutions mirrors the medical community's evolving approach to weight management. While previous generations relied on stimulants and appetite suppressants that often carried serious health risks, today's medications represent the culmination of decades of research into human metabolism, hormone function, and the complex interplay between body systems that influence weight. Modern treatments target specific biological pathways, working with the body's natural systems rather than fighting against them. This evolution hasn't just changed how we treat weight issues - it's transformed our entire understanding of obesity itself.

Looking ahead, this chapter will explore:

- The historical progression of weight loss medications and their impact on public health
- Key scientific breakthroughs that revolutionized our understanding of weight management
- The emergence of GLP-1 agonists and their role in modern obesity treatment
- Lessons learned from past approaches and how they inform current practices

As we examine this evolution, we'll see how each phase of development has contributed to our current understanding, helping to shape safer, more effective approaches to weight management. This history isn't just about the medications themselves - it's about our growing recognition of obesity as a complex medical condition requiring sophisticated, evidence-based solutions.

The significance of this progression extends beyond medical advancement. It represents a fundamental shift in how we approach weight management, moving from simplistic 'quick fixes' to comprehensive treatment strategies that consider the whole person. This transformation has opened new possibilities for millions struggling with weight management, offering hope through evidence-based solutions rather than dangerous shortcuts.

The Rise and Fall of Early Diet Pills: Understanding Historical Approaches

The history of diet pills serves as a sobering reminder of how desperation for quick weight loss solutions can lead down dangerous paths. In my mother's medicine cabinet, I once found an old amber bottle of diet pills from the 1960s, its faded label warning of side effects that would terrify any modern reader. This discovery sparked my interest in understanding how weight loss medication evolved from potentially lethal quick fixes to today's science-based solutions.

The early era of diet pills was marked by several concerning approaches:

- Amphetamine-based medications that promised rapid weight loss while causing dangerous side effects
- Thyroid hormone treatments prescribed to speed up metabolism, regardless of thyroid function
- DNP (2,4-Dinitrophenol) pills that increased metabolic rate but could cause fatal overheating
- Rainbow pills combining multiple stimulants with potentially deadly results

The 1960s and early 1970s saw the peak of amphetamine-based diet pill usage, with millions of Americans taking these medications despite mounting evidence of their dangers. These pills worked primarily by suppressing appetite and increasing energy, but they came with severe risks, including addiction, heart problems, and psychological disturbances.

Key warning signs that characterized dangerous early diet pills:

- Promises of unrealistic rapid weight loss
- Claims of "miracle" results without lifestyle changes
- Minimal or no medical oversight required
- Unknown or undisclosed ingredients
- Aggressive marketing targeting vulnerable populations

As I sorted through my mother's old diet pill collection, I found her handwritten notes describing the side effects she experienced - racing heart, sleepless nights, and anxiety. These personal accounts mirror the documented experiences of countless others who sought solutions through these early medications. Today, we understand that sustainable weight management requires a more nuanced approach than simply suppressing appetite or boosting metabolism at any cost.

For those considering weight loss medication today, the history of diet pills offers important lessons:

- Be wary of treatments promising unrealistic results
- Ensure any medication is FDA-approved and prescribed by a qualified healthcare provider
- Understand that effective weight management typically requires a comprehensive approach
- Research the documented safety profile of any medication you're considering
- Report any concerning side effects to your healthcare provider immediately

Perhaps the most notorious chapter in diet pill history came in the 1990s with the Fen-Phen combination. This drug pairing promised remarkable weight loss results but was ultimately pulled from the market after being linked to serious heart valve problems. The Fen-Phen disaster marked a turning point in weight loss medication development, leading to stricter FDA oversight and a renewed focus on safety in weight management treatments.

As a direct result of the lessons learned in this era, today's weight loss medications undergo rigorous testing, require proper medical supervision, and target specific biological pathways rather than simply stimulating the central nervous system. This evolution reflects our growing understanding of obesity as a complex medical condition requiring thoughtful, evidence-based treatment approaches.

The rise and fall of early diet pills serves as more than just a cautionary tale - it represents a crucial turning point in medical history. This evolution has led us to today's more sophisticated understanding of weight management, where safety and scientific evidence guide treatment decisions rather than quick-fix promises.

As we continue to advance in our understanding of obesity and weight management, the lessons learned from the early diet pill era remain relevant. They remind us that true progress in medical treatment comes not from seeking magic bullets but from patience, scientific investigation, and a commitment to safety above all else.

Breakthrough Science: How Understanding Gut Hormones Changed Everything

While organizing my home office last month, I found my old food diary from before starting weight loss medication. The detailed notes about constant hunger and cravings stood in stark contrast to my experience after beginning treatment. This personal transformation reflects a broader scientific breakthrough - understanding how our digestive system communicates with our brain to control hunger and satiety.

A key breakthrough came with the discovery of gut hormones that play crucial roles in appetite and metabolism:

- GLP-1 (Glucagon-like peptide-1): Signals fullness to the brain and slows stomach emptying
- PYY (Peptide YY): Reduces appetite and food intake
- Ghrelin: Known as the 'hunger hormone' that stimulates appetite
- CCK (Cholecystokinin): Released after eating to promote feelings of fullness

This understanding of gut hormones revealed why traditional dieting often fails. When we restrict calories, our bodies respond by increasing ghrelin and decreasing satiety hormones, creating a biological drive to eat more. This isn't about willpower - it's about powerful biological signals that evolved to protect us from starvation.

The impact of this scientific breakthrough extends beyond just understanding how our bodies regulate weight. It opened new possibilities for treatment by targeting these natural hormone pathways. Instead of fighting against the body's systems, modern medications work with them, mimicking or enhancing natural satiety signals.

During my first month using a GLP-1 agonist, I experienced firsthand how these hormones affect eating behavior. The constant mental calculations about food and portion sizes began to fade. For the first time, I could trust my body's signals about hunger and fullness. This wasn't just about eating less - it was about restoring normal appetite regulation that had been disrupted.

Understanding gut hormones has led to several important insights for weight management:

- Meal timing matters: Our hormone levels naturally fluctuate throughout the day
- Protein and fiber affect satiety hormone release
- Stress can disrupt normal hormone signaling
- Sleep quality impacts hunger hormone levels
- Regular exercise helps regulate appetite hormones

For anyone considering weight loss medication, understanding this gut hormone science helps explain both how the medications work and why they're more effective than previous approaches. Rather than simply suppressing appetite, these medications help restore normal hormone signaling patterns.

The practical implications of this breakthrough extend to daily habits that can support healthy hormone function:

- Eat protein with every meal to promote satiety
- Maintain consistent meal timing
- Prioritize adequate sleep

- Manage stress levels
- Include fiber-rich foods in your diet
- Stay hydrated throughout the day

This scientific understanding has transformed how we approach weight management. Instead of viewing excess weight as simply a matter of calories in versus calories out, we now recognize the complex hormonal orchestra that regulates appetite and metabolism. This shift has led to more effective treatments and a more compassionate understanding of why weight loss can be so challenging.

The breakthrough in understanding gut hormones also explains why some previous weight loss approaches were doomed to fail. Crash diets and extreme calorie restrictions work against our natural hormone systems, triggering biological responses that make sustained weight loss nearly impossible. Modern approaches based on hormone science offer a more sustainable path.

Looking ahead, this understanding continues to drive innovation in weight management treatment. New medications targeting multiple hormone pathways are in development, promising even more effective options for those struggling with weight management. This evolution in treatment options reflects our growing appreciation for the complexity of appetite regulation and weight control.

Modern Evolution: The Development and Impact of GLP-1 Agonists

The development of GLP-1 agonists represents one of the most significant breakthroughs in modern medicine's approach to weight management. Sitting at my kitchen table one morning, I noticed something remarkable - for the first time in decades, I had naturally stopped eating when I felt full, leaving half my breakfast untouched. This simple moment illustrated the profound impact these medications can have on our relationship with food.

GLP-1 agonists emerged from our growing understanding of how the body naturally regulates appetite and metabolism. These medications mimic the effects of our body's natural GLP-1 hormone, which plays several crucial roles:

- Slowing stomach emptying to help you feel full longer
- Reducing appetite by acting on brain centers that control hunger
- Improving insulin sensitivity and blood sugar control
- Decreasing inflammation throughout the body
- Supporting heart health through multiple mechanisms

The journey from discovery to widespread use of GLP-1 agonists showcases the evolution of modern weight management medicine. Initially developed for diabetes treatment, researchers noticed that patients taking these medications experienced significant weight loss. This observation led to further studies and eventually, the development of higher-dose versions specifically for weight management.

My personal experience with Zepbound reflects what many patients report - a fundamentally different experience from previous weight loss attempts. The medication doesn't just suppress appetite; it helps restore normal eating patterns and improves metabolic health. During my first month of treatment, I noticed several changes:

- Natural portion control without constant mental effort
- Reduced cravings for high-calorie foods
- Better blood sugar stability throughout the day
- Improved energy levels and mood
- Gradual, sustainable weight loss

The impact of GLP-1 agonists extends beyond individual success stories. These medications have challenged our traditional understanding of obesity treatment and opened new possibilities for managing weight-related health conditions. They've shown us that effective weight management isn't just about willpower - it's about addressing the biological factors that regulate appetite and metabolism.

For those considering GLP-1 agonists, several factors warrant consideration:

- Medical history and current health status
- Commitment to long-term treatment
- Insurance coverage and cost considerations
- Readiness to make complementary lifestyle changes
- Understanding of potential side effects

The success of GLP-1 agonists has sparked a new wave of research and development in weight management medicine. Scientists are now exploring combination therapies and new delivery methods that could make these treatments even more effective and accessible.

Perhaps most importantly, these medications have helped reshape the conversation around obesity treatment. Rather than viewing excess weight as a personal failing, we're increasingly recognizing it as a complex medical condition that often requires comprehensive medical intervention.

The development of GLP-1 agonists has also highlighted the importance of individualized treatment approaches. While these medications can be remarkably effective, they work best as part of a comprehensive weight management strategy that includes:

- Regular medical monitoring
- Dietary modifications
- Physical activity
- Stress management
- Adequate sleep
- Social support

Looking ahead, the impact of GLP-1 agonists continues to grow. New research is exploring their potential benefits beyond weight loss, including effects on cardiovascular health, mood disorders, and aging-related conditions. This ongoing evolution suggests we're still in the early stages of understanding the full potential of these remarkable medications.

The success of GLP-1 agonists has also catalyzed broader changes in healthcare delivery. More insurance companies are beginning to cover these medications, recognizing that effective weight management can prevent numerous costly health complications. Healthcare providers are developing specialized protocols for monitoring and supporting patients on these medications, ensuring optimal outcomes.

As we continue to learn more about GLP-1 agonists and their effects, one thing becomes increasingly clear: these medications represent not just a treatment option, but a paradigm shift in how we approach weight management. They've shown us that sustainable weight loss is possible when we work with, rather than against, our body's natural systems. As we conclude this journey through the evolution of weight loss medicine, it's clear that we've come remarkably far from the dangerous diet pills of yesteryear to today's sophisticated hormone-based treatments. This transformation mirrors our growing understanding of obesity as a complex medical condition rather than a simple matter of willpower.

For readers considering weight loss medication, consider these action steps:

- Research the historical context of any weight loss treatment you're considering
- Discuss your complete medical history with healthcare providers
- Understand both the benefits and risks of modern medications
- Develop realistic expectations based on scientific evidence rather than marketing claims

Looking ahead to the next chapter, we'll delve deeper into the science behind modern weight loss medications, exploring how they work with your body's natural systems to promote sustainable weight management. This understanding will provide crucial context for making informed decisions about your own weight management journey.

The story of weight loss medicine isn't just about the past - it's about building a future where safe and effective treatments are available to those who need them. As we've seen through this chapter, each step in this evolution has brought us closer to understanding the complex nature of weight management and developing more effective solutions.

Remember, whether you're considering weight loss medication or simply trying to understand the options available, knowledge of this history provides valuable context for making informed decisions. The lessons learned from past approaches continue to influence modern treatment strategies, helping ensure safer and more effective solutions for future generations.

2 BREAKING DOWN THE SCIENCE: HOW MODERN WEIGHT LOSS DRUGS TRANSFORM METABOLISM

The human body's metabolism is an intricate symphony of hormones, enzymes, and cellular processes that would put the most sophisticated orchestra to shame. Understanding how modern weight loss medications conduct this metabolic symphony is crucial for anyone considering these treatments as part of their weight management journey. Just as each instrument in an orchestra plays a vital role in creating beautiful music, each hormone and metabolic process in our body works in concert to regulate weight, appetite, and energy use. Understanding these intricate biological mechanisms has revolutionized how we approach weight management through medication.

During my first month on Zepbound, I decided to document the subtle changes in my body's response to food. As a lifelong cooking enthusiast who had always struggled with portion control, I was skeptical about how medication could change my relationship with food. I started keeping a detailed journal, noting not just what I ate but how my body responded. The transformation was fascinating - foods I once craved lost their magnetic pull, and my usual portion sizes suddenly felt overwhelming. One evening, while preparing my favorite pasta dish, I found myself doing something unprecedented: leaving food on my plate without any conscious effort. It wasn't about willpower anymore; my body was actually sending different signals. This personal experiment became a turning point in my understanding of how these medications work - not through forcing changes but by helping restore natural appetite signals that had long been disrupted.

This chapter will demystify the complex science behind modern weight loss medications, breaking down how they interact with our body's natural systems. We'll explore:

- How GLP-1 agonists communicate with your brain's appetite control center
- The role of gut hormones in regulating hunger and satiety
- How these medications affect your body's insulin sensitivity and glucose regulation

By understanding these mechanisms, you'll be better equipped to work with your healthcare provider to determine if these medications might be right for you. More importantly, you'll gain insight into why traditional approaches to weight loss often fall short and how modern medications can help bridge the gap between intention and action in weight management.

The journey through our body's metabolic processes reveals an amazing story of adaptation and balance. When we introduce weight loss medications into this system, we're not fighting against our body's natural processes - we're working to restore and optimize them. This understanding transformed my own approach to weight management, helping me see these medications not as a magic solution but as sophisticated tools that work in harmony with our body's natural systems.

As we explore the science behind these medications, you'll discover how they affect everything from brain chemistry to digestive processes, creating a comprehensive approach to weight management that extends far beyond simple calorie reduction. This knowledge will empower you to make informed decisions about your own weight management journey, understanding not just what these medications do but how they work with your body's natural systems to create sustainable change.

The GLP-1 Effect: Understanding Incretin Hormones and Appetite Control

Imagine your body has an intricate messaging system that helps regulate hunger, similar to a sophisticated thermostat that maintains the perfect temperature in your home. At the center of this system are incretin hormones, particularly GLP-1 (Glucagon-Like Peptide-1), which play a crucial role in how we experience hunger and fullness. Understanding how GLP-1 works has revolutionized our approach to weight management and explains why medications targeting this hormone have become so effective.

When we eat, our intestines naturally release GLP-1, triggering several important responses:

- Slowing down stomach emptying to help us feel full longer
- Reducing appetite signals in the brain
- Helping regulate blood sugar by stimulating insulin release
- Decreasing glucagon, a hormone that raises blood sugar

In many people struggling with obesity, this natural GLP-1 system isn't functioning optimally. It's like having a thermostat that's been miscalibrated - the signals aren't being sent or received correctly. This is where GLP-1 medications come into play, helping to restore these natural appetite control mechanisms.

During my first weeks on Zepbound, I experienced this hormone effect firsthand. Previously, I could easily finish a large restaurant portion without feeling satisfied. But now, I noticed a profound change in how my body responded to food. The medication wasn't forcing me to eat less - instead, it was helping my body recognize and respond to natural fullness signals that had long been muted.

The science behind GLP-1's effectiveness lies in its multi-targeted approach. Unlike older weight loss medications that simply tried to suppress appetite, GLP-1 agonists work with your body's natural systems in several ways:

- Enhancing the feeling of fullness after meals
- Reducing the urgency of hunger signals
- Improving blood sugar control
- Slowing digestion to maintain satiety longer

This comprehensive approach explains why many people report not just eating less, but experiencing a fundamental shift in their relationship with food. It's not about fighting against hunger - it's about restoring natural appetite regulation.

One evening, while preparing dinner, I realized how profoundly this medication had changed my eating patterns. Instead of mindlessly snacking while cooking, I found myself naturally waiting for the meal. The constant background hunger that had been my companion for years had transformed into clear, manageable hunger signals. This wasn't about willpower - it was about my body's messaging system finally working as intended.

For those considering GLP-1 medications, understanding this hormone effect can help set realistic expectations. These medications don't create artificial barriers to eating; rather, they help restore natural appetite control mechanisms that may have become dysregulated. This explains why the effects feel more natural and sustainable compared to traditional diet approaches.

Key indicators that your GLP-1 medication is working effectively include:

- Feeling satisfied with smaller portions
- Experiencing less urgent hunger between meals
- Having reduced interest in emotional eating
- Feeling more in control of food choices

However, it's important to remember that while GLP-1 medications can help restore these natural signals, they work best when supported by healthy eating habits and regular physical activity. The medication provides the biological support, but sustainable success comes from working with these restored signals to establish healthy, long-term habits.

As we continue to understand more about how incretin hormones influence our metabolism and eating behaviors, new medications and treatment approaches are being developed. This growing knowledge has opened up exciting possibilities for more effective and personalized weight management solutions, making it an encouraging time for those struggling with weight management to explore medical options.

Metabolic Mechanisms: How Weight Loss Drugs Affect Energy Processing

Understanding how weight loss medications affect our body's energy processing is like learning how to optimize a car's fuel efficiency. Just as a well-tuned engine converts fuel into energy more effectively, these medications help our bodies process and utilize energy from food more efficiently. Through my experience with Zepbound, I've gained firsthand insight into these intricate metabolic changes, and I'm excited to share how these medications influence our body's energy systems.

At its core, metabolism involves several key processes that weight loss medications can influence, including:

- Converting food into usable energy
- Storing excess energy as fat
- Breaking down stored fat for energy use
- Regulating blood sugar levels
- Controlling cellular energy expenditure

Modern weight loss medications work by influencing these processes in multiple ways, creating a more efficient metabolic environment for weight loss. When I first started my medication journey, I noticed changes not just in my appetite, but in my energy levels and how my body responded to different foods.

One morning, about six weeks into my treatment, I realized something remarkable while reviewing my food and energy journal. Despite eating fewer calories, I wasn't experiencing the afternoon energy crashes that had previously sent me searching for sugary snacks. This observation led me to deeper research into how these medications affect our cellular energy processing.

Weight loss medications can influence your metabolism in several important ways:

- Enhancing insulin sensitivity, helping cells better utilize glucose

- Increasing the breakdown of stored fat for energy
- Improving metabolic flexibility (the ability to switch between using carbs and fats for fuel)
- Reducing inflammation that can interfere with healthy metabolism
- Optimizing mitochondrial function for better energy production

These metabolic changes don't happen overnight. Think of it like gradually adjusting your home's thermostat - small changes lead to significant energy savings over time. The medications work to reset your body's metabolic thermostat to a more efficient setting.

During my third month on the medication, I noticed my body becoming more efficient at using stored energy. Previously, missing a meal would leave me shaky and irritable. Now, I found myself able to maintain steady energy levels even when my eating schedule varied. This wasn't just about eating less - it was about my body becoming better at accessing and using its stored energy reserves.

For those considering weight loss medication, understanding these metabolic mechanisms can help you:

- Recognize normal changes in energy levels during treatment
- Identify signs that your metabolism is responding to the medication
- Make dietary choices that support metabolic efficiency
- Time your meals and activities for optimal energy use
- Monitor your progress beyond just the scale

It's important to note that while these medications can significantly improve metabolic efficiency, they work best when supported by healthy lifestyle choices. Regular physical activity, adequate sleep, and proper nutrition all play crucial roles in optimizing your body's energy processing systems.

One of the most fascinating aspects of these medications is how they can help break the cycle of metabolic adaptation that often defeats traditional diet attempts. When we typically reduce calories, our bodies tend to compensate by slowing metabolism. Modern weight loss medications help maintain metabolic efficiency even as we consume fewer calories, making sustainable weight loss more achievable.

To maximize the metabolic benefits of these medications, consider implementing these strategies:

- Eat protein-rich meals to support muscle maintenance
- Include regular strength training in your exercise routine
- Stay well-hydrated to support metabolic processes
- Maintain consistent meal timing when possible
- Get adequate sleep to support hormonal balance

Through understanding how these medications influence our metabolism, we can work more effectively with our bodies rather than against them. This knowledge has transformed my approach to weight management, helping me make choices that support rather than hinder my body's natural energy processing systems.

Remember, while weight loss medications can significantly improve metabolic efficiency, they're not magic pills that override the fundamental principles of energy balance. Instead, they help create an internal environment where maintaining a healthy weight becomes more achievable, working with your body's natural systems rather than fighting against them.

Brain-Gut Connection: Neural Pathways in Modern Weight Loss Medication

Have you ever experienced butterflies in your stomach before a big presentation, or felt nauseous during times of stress? These sensations aren't just coincidences - they're direct evidence of the fascinating communication highway between your brain and gut, often called the gut-brain axis. This intricate connection plays a crucial role in how modern weight loss medications work, creating a harmonious dialogue between your digestive system and brain to regulate appetite and eating behaviors.

My own revelation about this connection came during a quiet Sunday morning breakfast. Three months into taking Zepbound, I noticed something remarkable - the persistent thoughts about food that used to occupy my mind had transformed into clear, manageable hunger signals. This wasn't just about feeling less hungry; it was about my brain and gut finally speaking the same language.

The brain-gut connection operates through several key pathways:

- The vagus nerve, our body's primary communication channel between brain and digestive system
- Neurotransmitters produced in both the brain and gut
- Hormone signals that regulate hunger and satiety
- Inflammatory markers that influence appetite and metabolism

Modern weight loss medications work by enhancing and optimizing these communication pathways. They help restore what I like to call your body's 'natural GPS' - guiding you back to more natural eating patterns by improving the signals between your gut and brain.

Think of your brain-gut connection like a sophisticated text messaging system. In many people struggling with weight, this messaging system has become cluttered with spam - false hunger signals, stress-eating triggers, and confused satiety cues. Weight loss medications help clean up this communication channel, ensuring that real hunger and fullness messages get through clearly.

To optimize your brain-gut connection while on weight loss medication, consider these practical strategies:

- Practice mindful eating by removing distractions during meals

- Keep a food-mood journal to track how different foods affect your mental state
- Allow 20 minutes for your brain to register fullness signals from your gut
- Stay hydrated to support optimal nerve signal transmission
- Manage stress through regular relaxation practices

One evening, while preparing dinner with my daughter, I experienced a profound example of this improved brain-gut communication. Instead of my usual anxious relationship with meal preparation, I found myself naturally attuned to my body's signals. The medication hadn't just reduced my appetite; it had helped restore my body's natural ability to regulate food intake.

Understanding this connection can help you recognize signs that your medication is working effectively. Some signs that your medication is working include:

- Reduced preoccupation with food between meals
- More consistent energy levels throughout the day
- Better ability to distinguish between emotional and physical hunger
- Improved satisfaction with smaller portions
- Natural meal spacing without clock-watching

The brain-gut connection also explains why weight loss medications often lead to changes in food preferences. Many people report naturally gravitating toward healthier foods - not because they're forcing themselves, but because their brain and gut are finally working together to signal what their body truly needs.

For those considering weight loss medication, understanding this neural pathway connection can help you:

- Set realistic expectations about how the medication will feel

- Recognize positive changes in your eating patterns
- Work with rather than against your body's natural signals
- Make informed decisions about timing meals and medication
- Identify when to seek adjustments in your treatment plan

Remember that while these medications can significantly improve brain-gut communication, they work best when supported by lifestyle habits that promote this connection. Regular exercise, adequate sleep, and stress management all play crucial roles in maintaining healthy neural pathways.

Through my journey with weight loss medication, I've come to appreciate how this restored brain-gut connection extends beyond just managing my weight - it's about reestablishing a harmonious relationship with food and our bodies. When our internal communication systems work properly, making healthy choices becomes less about willpower and more about listening to our body's natural wisdom. As we conclude our exploration of the science behind modern weight loss medications, it's clear that these treatments represent far more than just appetite suppressants - they are sophisticated tools that work in harmony with our body's natural systems. Understanding these mechanisms transforms how we view weight management, moving from simplistic 'eat less, move more' approaches to recognizing the complex interplay of hormones, neural pathways, and metabolic processes.

The journey through your body's metabolic landscape can feel overwhelming, but let's distill what we've learned into actionable insights:

- Your body's appetite control system operates like a finely tuned thermostat, with GLP-1 playing a crucial role in regulating hunger and fullness
- Modern weight loss medications work by enhancing natural processes rather than fighting against them

- The brain-gut connection forms a crucial communication highway that these medications help optimize
- Metabolic efficiency improves gradually, similar to fine-tuning an engine for better performance

For anyone considering weight loss medication, these key takeaways can help guide your decision-making process:

- Work with your healthcare provider to understand how these medications might interact with your unique body chemistry
- Monitor not just weight changes, but also shifts in energy levels, appetite patterns, and food preferences
- Prepare for gradual changes in how your body processes and responds to food
- Consider keeping a journal to track your body's responses and communicate effectively with your healthcare team

My own experience with Zepbound taught me that success with these medications isn't just about the numbers on the scale - it's about understanding and working with your body's natural systems. That morning when I first left food on my plate without effort wasn't just about eating less; it represented a fundamental shift in how my body communicated its needs.

Looking ahead, this understanding of metabolic mechanisms opens new possibilities for personalized approaches to weight management. Just as we've moved from one-size-fits-all diets to recognizing individual metabolic differences, our growing knowledge of how these medications work allows for more targeted and effective treatments.

Remember, while science has given us powerful tools for weight management, true success comes from working with, rather than against, our body's natural processes. These medications don't override our biology - they help restore and optimize systems that may have become unbalanced over time.

As you continue your own weight management journey, let this deeper understanding of metabolic mechanisms guide your decisions and expectations. Whether you choose to incorporate medication into your weight management plan or not, knowing how your body works helps you make more informed choices about your health and well-being.

3 THE BIG PLAYERS: UNDERSTANDING OZEMPIC, WEGOVY, ZEPBOUND, AND BEYOND

Standing in my doctor's office last year, I faced a decision that millions of Americans are now confronting: choosing between several powerful weight loss medications that each offered unique benefits and considerations. The landscape of weight loss medication has evolved dramatically, with Ozempic, Wegovy, and Zepbound emerging as revolutionary tools that work in subtly different ways to address weight management.

This new era of pharmaceutical weight management has ushered in unprecedented options, each with its own unique benefits and considerations. As we explore these medications in detail, it's essential to understand not just how they work, but also their distinct characteristics that make them suitable for different individuals and situations.

The waiting room at my doctor's office was unusually quiet that Tuesday morning as I prepared for my monthly check-in. After six months on Zepbound, I had lost 42 pounds, but more importantly, I had gained a new understanding of how these medications worked. As I sat there, I noticed three other patients, each at different stages of their weight loss journey.

Maria, a nurse I'd met during previous visits, was starting Wegovy after careful consideration. Tom, a retired teacher, had been on Ozempic for diabetes management and experienced significant weight loss as a beneficial side effect. And Amy, newly prescribed Zepbound, was eagerly asking questions about what to expect. As we shared our experiences, it struck me how each of our journeys was unique yet connected by these innovative medications.

Our conversation revealed the various factors that led each of us to choose different medications - from insurance coverage to specific health conditions to lifestyle considerations. This impromptu support group in the waiting room perfectly illustrated how these different medications serve diverse needs in the weight management landscape and why having multiple options is so crucial for personalized treatment approaches.

Understanding these medications requires more than just knowing their names or basic functions. It's about grasping how each option might fit into your particular health journey, considering factors like your medical history, lifestyle, and weight loss goals. This knowledge becomes particularly crucial as more medications enter the market and treatment options continue to expand.

The landscape of weight loss medication has evolved dramatically in recent years, with each new development bringing both excitement and questions. For many, the abundance of options can feel overwhelming. However, this variety actually represents a significant advantage - it means there's a greater chance of finding a medication that aligns perfectly with your individual needs and circumstances.

In this chapter, we'll examine the key players in the modern weight loss medication landscape, breaking down their similarities and differences in ways that matter to you as a potential patient.

We'll explore:

- The specific mechanisms that make each medication unique
- Real-world effectiveness and typical results
- Cost considerations and insurance coverage
- Dosing schedules and administration methods
- FDA-approved uses and off-label applications
- Long-term usage considerations

By the end of this chapter, you'll have a clear understanding of how these medications compare, helping you make more informed decisions about your weight management journey in partnership with your healthcare provider.

Comparing the Giants: Ozempic vs. Wegovy vs. Zepbound - Understanding Key Differences

Let me share a moment that crystallized the differences between these medications for me. While organizing my home office, I came across three distinct medication information packets - one each for Ozempic, Wegovy, and Zepbound. Though they might seem similar at first glance, each serves a unique purpose in the weight management landscape.

These medications share a common foundation as GLP-1 receptor agonists, but they have distinct characteristics that set them apart:

Ozempic (semaglutide)

- Primary FDA approval for Type 2 diabetes management
- Weekly injection with doses ranging from 0.25mg to 2mg
- Often prescribed off-label for weight loss
- Typically lower cost due to diabetes coverage

Wegovy (semaglutide)

- Specifically FDA-approved for chronic weight management
- Higher dose range than Ozempic (up to 2.4mg weekly)
- More likely to be covered by insurance for weight loss
- Same active ingredient as Ozempic but different dosing protocol

Zepbound (tirzepatide)

- Newest to market for weight management
- Different active ingredient than semaglutide
- Targets both GLP-1 and GIP receptors
- Potentially stronger weight loss effects in clinical trials

Understanding these differences became crucial in my own journey. After discussing options with my healthcare provider, we chose Zepbound because of its dual-action mechanism and my specific health profile. The decision wasn't just about which medication might work best, but also considered practical factors like insurance coverage, dosing schedule, and potential side effects.

When comparing these medications, several key factors should guide your decision-making process:

- Medical history and current health status
- Presence of diabetes or pre-diabetes
- Previous medication experiences
- Other health conditions
- Current medications
- Practical considerations
- Insurance coverage and cost
- Injection schedule preference
- Support from healthcare provider
- Access to medication

The effectiveness of these medications can vary significantly among individuals. While Zepbound has shown slightly higher average weight loss in clinical trials, this doesn't necessarily mean it's the best choice for everyone. Your body's response, tolerance for side effects, and personal health goals all play crucial roles in determining the most appropriate medication.

I've found that tracking specific aspects of each medication can help in discussions with your healthcare provider:

- Weekly weight changes
- Side effect experiences
- Appetite patterns
- Energy levels
- Medication costs and coverage

Remember that these medications aren't interchangeable, despite their similarities. Each has its own unique protocol for starting and adjusting doses. For instance, Wegovy follows a specific five-step dose escalation process, while Zepbound has its own distinct titration schedule. These differences in dosing strategies can impact both effectiveness and side effect management.

One crucial aspect often overlooked is the transition between medications. If you're considering switching from one to another, it's essential to work closely with your healthcare provider to develop a proper transition plan. This might involve a gradual tapering off one medication before starting another, or specific timing considerations to maintain effectiveness while minimizing side effects.

The choice between these medications often comes down to a combination of medical necessity, practical considerations, and personal preferences. Your healthcare provider will consider factors such as:

- Your BMI and weight loss goals
- Presence of weight-related conditions
- Previous weight loss attempts
- Insurance coverage and cost considerations
- Your comfort with injection schedules
- Potential drug interactions

As you consider these options, maintain open communication with your healthcare provider about your preferences and concerns. Document your questions and observations about each medication to facilitate more productive discussions during your appointments. Remember, the 'best' medication is the one that aligns with your specific needs, circumstances, and health goals while being practically sustainable for your lifestyle.

Beyond the Basics: Dosing, Duration, and Expected Outcomes

The morning I started my weight loss medication journey, I carefully reviewed the dosing instructions, wondering how this would fit into my daily routine. Like many others, I had questions about what to expect: How long would it take to see results? What was the right dose for me? How would I know if the medication was working? These questions reflect common concerns that deserve clear, practical answers.

Understanding the basics of dosing and duration is crucial for success with weight loss medications. Most modern weight loss medications follow a gradual dose escalation schedule to help your body adjust and minimize side effects. Here's what you need to know about typical dosing patterns:

- Starting doses are usually lower than therapeutic doses
- Dose increases typically occur every 4 weeks
- Full therapeutic doses are usually reached within 4-5 months
- Regular monitoring with your healthcare provider guides dose adjustments
- Some patients may need longer at certain doses before advancing

My own experience with Zepbound taught me the importance of patience during the dose escalation period. The first month at a lower dose allowed my body to adjust gradually, minimizing side effects while still seeing initial results. Each dose increase brought new adjustments, but also increased effectiveness.

When it comes to expected outcomes, it's important to set realistic expectations based on clinical evidence. While individual results vary, most people can expect:

- Initial weight loss within the first month
- More significant results by months 3-6

- Maximum effectiveness usually seen by month 6
- Continued results with maintained use
- Potential plateau periods requiring dose adjustments

Tracking your progress becomes essential during this journey. I developed a simple monitoring system that included:

- Weekly weigh-ins at the same time
- Notes about appetite changes and food preferences
- Side effect documentation
- Energy level observations
- Monthly measurements beyond just weight

The duration of treatment varies significantly among individuals. Some may need only 6-12 months of medication support, while others benefit from longer-term use. Your healthcare provider will help determine the appropriate duration based on your progress and health goals.

One Sunday morning, six months into treatment, I reviewed my progress journal and noticed interesting patterns. The most significant changes weren't just in the numbers on the scale but in my daily habits and relationship with food. The medication had created a window of opportunity for developing sustainable lifestyle changes.

To optimize your outcomes, consider these practical strategies:

- Take your medication at the same time each day or week
- Keep a detailed log of your progress and side effects
- Maintain regular communication with your healthcare provider
- Plan for dose adjustment periods
- Set realistic milestones for progress evaluation

Understanding the timing of results helps manage expectations. While some people see dramatic early results, others experience more gradual changes. The key is consistency and patience. Your body needs time to adjust to both the medication and the lifestyle changes it enables.

Regular monitoring becomes crucial for long-term success. Work with your healthcare provider to establish:

- Regular check-in schedules
- Clear criteria for dose adjustments
- Specific health markers to track
- Plans for addressing plateaus
- Strategies for maintaining results

Remember that the journey isn't just about the numbers on the scale. Success often appears in various forms, including:

- Improved energy levels
- Better sleep quality
- Changed eating habits
- Reduced cravings
- Enhanced mobility

Making informed decisions about dosing and duration requires open communication with your healthcare provider. Bring your concerns and questions to each appointment, and don't hesitate to discuss adjustments when needed. This collaborative approach ensures you're getting the most benefit from your medication while maintaining safety and effectiveness.

As you progress through your medication journey, stay focused on your personal goals while remaining flexible about the path to achieve them. The medication provides support, but your commitment to the process ultimately determines your success.

The Pipeline: Emerging Medications and Future Developments

Recently, while organizing my home office, I discovered a folder filled with articles about emerging weight loss treatments that I'd collected over the past year. The sheer volume of new developments was striking - a testament to the rapid evolution in this field. The future of weight loss medicine extends far beyond what's currently available, with promising new medications and innovative delivery systems on the horizon.

The pipeline of emerging weight loss medications is particularly exciting, with several noteworthy developments in clinical trials:

- Triple-hormone receptor medications that target GLP-1, GIP, and glucagon
- Once-monthly injection options for improved convenience
- Oral formulations of current injectable medications
- Combination therapies that pair existing medications with new compounds
- Smart delivery systems that adjust dosing based on individual response

One morning, while reviewing my own medication journey notes, I reflected on how different my experience might have been with some of these emerging technologies. The weekly injection routine that had become part of my life could potentially be replaced by a monthly visit or even a daily pill. These advances aren't just about convenience - they represent potential breakthroughs in how we approach weight management.

The development of new weight loss medications focuses on several key areas of innovation:

- Enhanced Effectiveness: Targeting multiple hormone pathways simultaneously

- Improved Delivery: Making administration easier and more convenient
- Reduced Side Effects: Developing formulations with better tolerability
- Personalized Medicine: Creating treatments tailored to individual responses
- Cost Efficiency: Working toward more affordable treatment options

During a recent telemedicine appointment, my doctor shared exciting news about a clinical trial for a new oral formulation of a GLP-1 agonist. The potential to switch from injections to pills could dramatically change how many people approach medical weight management. However, she emphasized that these developments, while promising, require thorough testing and regulatory approval before becoming available.

For those considering weight loss medication now or in the future, it's helpful to understand how to evaluate emerging treatments.

- Research the stage of clinical trials and expected timeline to market
- Consider waiting for newer options if current treatments aren't ideal
- Discuss upcoming medications with your healthcare provider
- Monitor FDA announcements about new approvals
- Stay informed about insurance coverage for new treatments

The landscape of weight loss medication is evolving rapidly, but this progress brings both opportunities and challenges. While new treatments offer exciting possibilities, they also require careful evaluation and consideration. As someone who has benefited from current medications, I'm optimistic about these developments while maintaining realistic expectations about their timeline and accessibility.

Practical considerations for staying informed about emerging treatments include:

- Following reputable medical news sources
- Joining patient advocacy groups
- Maintaining regular discussions with your healthcare provider
- Understanding the difference between approved treatments and those in development
- Considering participation in clinical trials if appropriate

The future of weight loss medicine extends beyond just new medications. Innovative approaches being developed include:

- AI-driven dosing systems
- Microbiome-based treatments
- Targeted genetic therapies
- Smart monitoring devices
- Integrated treatment platforms

As these new treatments move through the development pipeline, it's important to maintain perspective. While the promise of improved medications is exciting, current treatments continue to offer effective options for many people. The key is working with your healthcare provider to find the right solution for your needs, whether that's an existing medication or waiting for an emerging treatment that better suits your situation.

Remember that the development of new medications is a methodical process designed to ensure safety and effectiveness. While we may be excited about future possibilities, it's essential to focus on currently available, proven treatments while keeping an eye on emerging options that might better serve our needs in the future.

As we conclude our exploration of today's leading weight loss medications, it's clear that the landscape of medical weight management has evolved significantly. From my personal journey with Zepbound to the shared experiences of countless others using Ozempic and Wegovy, these medications represent more than just pharmaceutical innovations – they symbolize a new chapter in how we approach weight management.

Your journey with weight loss medication will be as unique as you are. Whether you're considering Ozempic for its dual benefit in diabetes management, Wegovy for its specialized weight loss protocol, or Zepbound for its innovative dual-hormone approach, success depends on making an informed choice that aligns with your specific needs and circumstances.

As you move forward, consider these action steps to help guide your decision:

- Schedule a comprehensive consultation with your healthcare provider
- Review your insurance coverage for each medication option
- Document your current health status and weight loss goals
- Consider your lifestyle and how each medication might fit into it
- Prepare questions about side effects and management strategies

Remember that choosing a weight loss medication is just the first step in your journey. The medication you start with may not be the one you stay with long-term, and that's okay. The goal is finding the right tool that works for your body, your lifestyle, and your health objectives.

In my own experience, the decision to start Zepbound came after careful consideration of all available options and honest discussions with my healthcare provider about my goals and concerns. This thoughtful approach to choosing the right medication has made all the difference in my success.

The key takeaways from this chapter highlight several crucial points for anyone considering these medications:

- Each medication has unique characteristics that may make it more suitable for specific individuals
- The choice of medication often depends on factors beyond just weight loss goals
- Insurance coverage and accessibility play significant roles in treatment decisions
- Regular medical monitoring and dose adjustments are essential for success
- Understanding potential side effects and management strategies is crucial

As we look ahead to discussing the real benefits and hidden risks of these medications in the next chapter, carry forward this understanding of the current market leaders. Your knowledge of these options will help you engage more effectively with your healthcare provider and make more informed decisions about your weight management journey.

The world of weight loss medication continues to evolve, but understanding today's options gives you the foundation needed to make educated choices about your health. Whether you choose Ozempic, Wegovy, Zepbound, or await future developments, the key is making an informed decision that aligns with your personal health journey.

4 BEYOND THE HYPE: REAL BENEFITS AND HIDDEN RISKS OF WEIGHT LOSS MEDICATIONS

Weight loss medications have become the subject of countless headlines, social media posts, and water cooler conversations, often blurring the line between fact and fiction. As both a researcher and someone who has experienced both the triumphs and challenges of these medications firsthand, I've witnessed how the promise of dramatic weight loss can sometimes overshadow important discussions about risks and realistic outcomes. The reality is that weight loss medications represent a powerful but complex medical intervention that requires careful consideration and honest evaluation.

Last summer, I attended a weight management support group where I met Rebecca, a successful accountant who had been on a GLP-1 agonist for eight months. She arrived at the meeting visibly frustrated, despite having lost 45 pounds. 'Everyone told me this would be easy,' she shared, describing how social media had painted these medications as miracle solutions. While her weight loss was significant, she had struggled with persistent nausea during the first three months and had to learn to navigate social situations with her changed relationship with food. Through careful medication management and lifestyle adjustments, she eventually found her balance. Rebecca's story became a powerful reminder of why I wrote this book - to help others understand that while these medications can be transformative, success requires realistic expectations, proper medical supervision, and a commitment to working through challenges. Her experience exemplifies the importance of understanding both the benefits and risks of weight loss medications, rather than falling for oversimplified promises.

The landscape of weight loss medication benefits can be broken down into several key areas:

- Clinically significant weight reduction
- Improved metabolic health markers
- Enhanced quality of life
- Better management of obesity-related conditions
- Increased mobility and physical function

However, these benefits come with important considerations that every potential user should understand. The journey with weight loss medications isn't always straightforward, and success often requires navigating various challenges while maintaining a balanced perspective.

Throughout this chapter, we'll examine the documented benefits of these medications through the lens of scientific evidence, while also taking an unflinching look at potential risks and side effects. We'll explore how different medications affect the body, what kind of results you can realistically expect, and what warning signs to watch for during treatment.

Most importantly, we'll discuss how to evaluate whether the potential benefits outweigh the risks for your specific situation. This includes understanding not just the physical impacts, but also the emotional and psychological aspects of treatment. By the end of this chapter, you'll have a clearer picture of what these medications can and cannot do, helping you make a more informed decision about your weight management journey.

The goal isn't to discourage anyone from considering these medications, but rather to ensure that those who choose this path do so with clear eyes and realistic expectations. After all, the most successful treatment outcomes often come from being well-informed and prepared for both the triumphs and challenges ahead.

Documented Benefits: Understanding Real-World Results and Success Rates

When evaluating weight loss medications, understanding real-world results beyond clinical trials provides crucial insights into what patients can realistically expect. Through my experience with Zepbound and extensive documentation of others' journeys, I've observed that success rates and benefits often manifest in multiple ways beyond just the numbers on the scale.

The most commonly reported benefits of modern weight loss medications include:

- Average weight loss of 10-15% of body weight within the first year
- Significant improvements in blood pressure and blood sugar levels
- Reduced joint pain and improved mobility
- Better sleep quality and increased energy levels
- Decreased food cravings and improved portion control

One morning, while reviewing my progress journal from the past year, I noticed how my success metrics had evolved. Initially, I focused solely on pounds lost, but as time went on I began tracking other meaningful changes - like being able to play with my grandchildren without getting winded, fitting comfortably in airplane seats, and maintaining stable blood sugar levels throughout the day. These real-world benefits often prove more meaningful than the raw numbers.

However, it's essential to understand that results vary significantly among individuals. While some patients experience dramatic transformations, others may see more modest changes. Factors influencing success rates include:

- Starting weight and overall health status
- Consistency with medication protocol
- Integration of lifestyle modifications
- Individual biological response to the medication
- Level of support and medical monitoring

During a support group meeting last month, I met Maria, who had been on a GLP-1 agonist for six months. Her success wasn't measured in pounds alone - though she had lost 40 pounds, the more significant victory was no longer needing blood pressure medication. This kind of comprehensive health improvement represents the true potential of these medications when used as part of a complete treatment approach.

Tracking your progress effectively can help you understand your personal response to the medication. Consider monitoring:

- Weekly weight measurements
- Monthly body measurements
- Changes in medication dosages for other conditions
- Energy levels and mood
- Physical activity capacity
- Food portion sizes and hunger signals

The key to interpreting success rates lies in understanding that weight loss medications work differently for each person. While clinical trials show impressive average results, real-world outcomes often tell a more nuanced story. Some patients experience rapid initial weight loss followed by a plateau, while others see steady, gradual progress over time.

My own journey with Zepbound taught me that success isn't linear. There were weeks of significant progress followed by periods of maintenance, and understanding this pattern helped me maintain realistic expectations. The medication provided consistent support in managing portion sizes and reducing cravings, but the rate of weight loss varied throughout the year.

Perhaps most importantly, documented benefits extend beyond physical changes. Many patients report improved relationships with food, reduced anxiety around eating, and better overall quality of life. These psychological benefits, while harder to measure, often prove just as valuable as the physical transformations.

When evaluating whether these medications might be right for you, consider creating a personal benefits checklist that includes both weight-related goals and other health objectives. This broader perspective can help you better assess the medication's impact on your overall wellbeing, not just the number on the scale.

Remember that success with weight loss medications isn't just about reaching a target weight - it's about achieving sustainable health improvements that enhance your quality of life. The most successful patients often view these medications as tools that support broader lifestyle changes rather than magical solutions working in isolation.

Hidden Risks: Common Side Effects and Long-Term Considerations

My first encounter with medication side effects came three weeks into starting Zepbound. Despite following all protocols carefully, I experienced unexpected nausea during a family dinner. This eye-opening experience taught me the importance of understanding not just the benefits, but also the potential risks and side effects of weight loss medications. While these medications can be transformative for many people, being well-informed about possible complications is crucial for making sound decisions about your health journey.

Common side effects of GLP-1 agonists and similar weight loss medications include:

- Gastrointestinal issues (nausea, vomiting, diarrhea)
- Headaches and fatigue
- Injection site reactions
- Changes in taste preferences
- Delayed gastric emptying

These initial side effects often occur during the first few weeks of treatment as your body adjusts to the medication. While many people find these symptoms manageable and temporary, others may need to work closely with their healthcare provider to find the right dosing strategy or consider alternative options.

More serious potential risks that require immediate medical attention include:

- Severe stomach pain
- Persistent vomiting
- Signs of pancreatitis
- Allergic reactions
- Significant changes in heart rate

During a recent support group meeting, I met Thomas, who shared his experience with managing side effects. He discovered that taking his medication at night and eating smaller, more frequent meals helped minimize his nausea. His story highlighted how personalized management strategies can make a significant difference in the medication experience.

Long-term considerations extend beyond immediate side effects. While these medications are relatively new, emerging research suggests several areas that require ongoing monitoring:

- Potential impact on bone density
- Effects on gallbladder function
- Changes in nutrient absorption
- Psychological adaptation to altered eating patterns
- Impact on medication interactions

To help monitor and manage potential risks, consider these practical steps:

- Keep a detailed symptom diary
- Schedule regular check-ups with your healthcare provider
- Monitor your vitamin and mineral levels
- Stay hydrated and maintain balanced nutrition

- Learn to recognize warning signs that require medical attention

My own experience taught me the value of preparation and proactive management. I developed a routine of taking my medication with evening meals and always keeping ginger tea and small protein snacks nearby. These simple strategies helped me navigate through the adjustment period successfully.

It's important to note that not everyone experiences significant side effects, and many find them manageable with proper support and guidance. However, understanding these risks allows you to make informed decisions and prepare appropriate management strategies.

When considering weight loss medications, ask yourself these key questions:

- Do I have access to regular medical monitoring?
- Am I prepared to manage potential side effects?
- Do I have a support system in place?
- Have I discussed potential medication interactions with my healthcare provider?
- Do I understand the warning signs that require immediate medical attention?

Remember that managing risks doesn't mean avoiding treatment altogether - it means approaching it with awareness and preparation. Success often comes from finding the right balance between managing side effects and maintaining commitment to your health goals.

One particularly important consideration is the long-term impact on eating behaviors and metabolism. While these medications can help establish healthier eating patterns, they're not meant to be a permanent solution for everyone. Understanding how your body might respond when discontinuing medication is crucial for long-term planning.

The key to successful risk management lies in maintaining open communication with your healthcare provider and being proactive about monitoring your body's responses. By staying informed and prepared, you can better navigate the challenges while maximizing the benefits of these medications.

Risk-Benefit Analysis: Tools for Making Informed Decisions

Making informed decisions about weight loss medications requires carefully weighing potential benefits against risks for your specific situation. As I sat at my kitchen table one evening, creating a decision matrix to evaluate whether Zepbound was right for me, I realized how valuable a structured approach to this decision could be for others facing the same choice.

A comprehensive risk-benefit analysis should consider these key areas:

- Your current health status and medical history
- Potential improvements in health markers and quality of life
- Possible side effects and their impact on daily activities
- Financial considerations and insurance coverage
- Available support systems and medical monitoring
- Alternative treatment options

To help you conduct your own analysis, I've developed a practical framework based on both personal experience and extensive research. Start by rating each factor on a scale of 1-5, with 5 representing the highest importance to you:

- Urgency of weight loss for health reasons
- Tolerance for potential side effects
- Financial ability to maintain treatment
- Access to medical support
- Impact on daily routine and lifestyle

- Long-term health implications

After completing my own analysis, I discovered that while the potential benefits of significant weight loss and improved blood pressure were compelling, I needed to carefully consider how the medication might affect my busy work schedule and family life. This systematic approach helped me make a more confident decision about starting treatment.

Consider creating a personal decision journal that tracks:

- Your primary motivations for considering medication
- Current health metrics and goals
- Potential lifestyle adjustments needed
- Support resources available
- Financial planning for treatment

One valuable tool I've found is the 'Week in the Life' exercise. Before starting medication, document a typical week in your life, including:

- Daily routines and meal patterns
- Work and family commitments
- Exercise habits and physical activities
- Social events and dining situations
- Stress levels and emotional eating triggers

This baseline assessment helps you anticipate how medication might impact your daily life and what adjustments you might need to make. During my first month on Zepbound, referring back to this exercise helped me identify which aspects of my routine needed modification to accommodate the medication's effects.

To make your risk-benefit analysis more concrete, consider these practical steps:

- Schedule a thorough medical evaluation

- Research your insurance coverage and out-of-pocket costs
- Identify potential lifestyle modifications needed
- Plan for possible side effect management
- Establish a support network
- Set realistic expectations and timeline goals

Remember that this decision isn't just about numbers on a scale. During my support group meetings, I've noticed how different individuals weigh various factors differently. Sarah, a busy executive, prioritized the medication's impact on her work performance, while Michael, a retiree with diabetes, focused more on long-term health benefits.

A thoughtful risk-benefit analysis should also consider your readiness for change. Ask yourself:

- Am I prepared to make necessary lifestyle adjustments?
- Do I have realistic expectations about outcomes?
- Can I commit to regular medical monitoring?
- Have I explored alternative weight management options?
- Do I understand the long-term implications of treatment?

The decision to start weight loss medication is deeply personal, but it shouldn't be made in isolation. Consulting with healthcare providers, family members, and others who have experience with these medications can provide valuable perspectives for your analysis.

Keep in mind that your initial decision isn't permanent. Regular reassessment of benefits and risks throughout your treatment journey helps ensure the medication continues to serve your health goals effectively. My own quarterly reviews have helped me adjust my treatment plan as needed and maintain a clear perspective on my progress.

By taking a systematic approach to evaluating benefits and risks, you can make a more confident decision about whether weight loss medication is right for you. Remember, the goal isn't to eliminate all risks but to make an informed choice that aligns with your health objectives and personal circumstances.As we conclude our exploration of the real benefits and hidden risks of weight loss medications, it's clear that success in this journey requires more than just understanding the medical facts - it requires a balanced perspective and realistic expectations.

Before moving forward with weight loss medications, consider these action steps:

- Schedule a comprehensive health evaluation with your healthcare provider
- Create a detailed list of your current medications and health conditions
- Document your weight loss history and previous treatment experiences
- Research your insurance coverage and financial options
- Identify your support system and resources for ongoing guidance

Remember Rebecca's story from the beginning of this chapter - her journey reminds us that while social media and marketing may paint an oversimplified picture, the reality of weight loss medication treatment is more nuanced. Success comes not from seeking a miracle solution, but from approaching these medications as powerful tools that require careful consideration and ongoing management.

Moving forward, use the risk-benefit analysis tools and decision-making frameworks we've discussed to evaluate your own situation. Consider how the potential benefits align with your health goals and how prepared you are to manage possible challenges. Remember that making an informed decision about weight loss medication isn't just about gathering information - it's about understanding how that information applies to your unique circumstances.

The key takeaways from this chapter include:

- Weight loss medications offer significant benefits when used appropriately and under proper medical supervision
- Understanding and preparing for side effects is crucial for long-term success
- Regular monitoring and open communication with healthcare providers are essential
- Individual responses to medications vary significantly
- Risk-benefit analysis should be personalized to each individual's situation

Whether you're just beginning to explore weight loss medications or are already on your treatment journey, maintaining realistic expectations while staying informed about both benefits and risks will serve you well. The path to successful weight management through medication isn't always straight or simple, but with proper preparation and understanding, it can be navigated successfully.

In the next chapter, we'll explore how to determine if you're a good candidate for weight loss medications, building on the foundation of knowledge we've established here about benefits and risks. This understanding will help you make more informed decisions about your weight management journey.

5 YOUR PERSONAL PRESCRIPTION: DETERMINING IF WEIGHT LOSS DRUGS ARE RIGHT FOR YOU

Making the decision to start weight loss medication isn't just about wanting to lose weight - it's about evaluating whether you're medically and personally ready for this significant step in your health journey.

As I sat in my doctor's office reviewing my health markers and discussing my weight loss goals, I realized that this decision required careful consideration of multiple factors—both medical and personal— that I hadn't previously thought about. What works brilliantly for one person may not be suitable for another, making this a deeply individual decision that deserves thorough evaluation.

As someone who has navigated this decision-making process myself, I understand the mix of hope, uncertainty, and questions that arise when considering weight loss medications. The landscape of modern weight management drugs offers promising options, but it also requires careful evaluation of your personal health profile, lifestyle readiness, and long-term goals.

Key factors to consider when evaluating if weight loss medications are right for you include:

- Current BMI and health status
- Previous weight loss attempts and outcomes
- Existing medical conditions and medications
- Lifestyle factors and daily routine
- Support system and resources
- Insurance coverage and financial considerations

The decision to start weight loss medication extends far beyond simply wanting to lose weight. It requires an honest assessment of your readiness for change and commitment to the journey ahead. This means being prepared for regular medical monitoring, potential lifestyle adjustments, and the dedication needed to make the most of these powerful tools.

My own decision process involved months of careful tracking, reflection, and discussion with healthcare providers. The detailed journal I kept of my weight loss history, medical markers, and health goals became invaluable during my initial consultation. This level of preparation not only impressed my doctor but also helped ensure I was making an informed decision aligned with my health objectives.

The turning point came during my consultation when reviewing my BMI of 32, my history of previous weight loss attempts, and my commitment to making lifestyle changes alongside medication use. Together with my healthcare provider, we examined how the medication would fit into my daily routine, considering my work schedule and family commitments. This thorough evaluation process laid the groundwork for what would become a successful weight management journey.

This chapter will guide you through your own decision-making process, providing practical tools and considerations to help you evaluate whether weight loss medication could be an appropriate part of your health journey. We'll explore the medical criteria, lifestyle factors, and personal considerations that should inform your choice, while addressing common concerns and questions that arise during this important decision process.

Remember, the goal isn't just to determine if you're eligible for weight loss medication, but to assess whether it's the right tool for your specific situation and goals. Through careful evaluation and honest self-assessment, you can make an informed decision that aligns with your health objectives and personal circumstances.

Medical Criteria and Personal Health Assessment: Understanding If You're a Candidate

Understanding if you're a candidate for weight loss medication involves evaluating several key medical criteria and personal health factors. When I first considered medication for weight management, I discovered that eligibility extends beyond simply wanting to lose weight - it requires meeting specific medical guidelines while also being in the right place personally to commit to treatment.

The primary medical criteria for weight loss medication candidacy typically include:

- A body mass index (BMI) of 30 or higher, or 27+ with weight-related health conditions
- A history of unsuccessful weight loss attempts through diet and exercise alone
- No contraindications or medical conditions that would make the medication unsafe
- Stable mental health and ability to follow treatment protocols
- No current pregnancy or plans to become pregnant

Beyond these basic criteria, healthcare providers will conduct a thorough health assessment that examines:

- Current medications and potential interactions
- Cardiovascular health and blood pressure
- Liver and kidney function
- Thyroid health and hormone levels
- History of eating disorders or substance abuse

During my initial health assessment, my doctor explained that meeting the medical criteria was just the first step. The evaluation process revealed aspects of my health I hadn't considered relevant to weight management. My slightly elevated blood pressure, for instance, became an important factor in monitoring my treatment progress.

The personal health assessment goes deeper than medical measurements, requiring honest reflection about your readiness for this journey. Consider these key questions:

- Are you prepared for regular medical check-ups and monitoring?

- Can you commit to following medication schedules and guidelines consistently?
- Do you have the support system needed for successful treatment?
- Are you willing to make concurrent lifestyle changes?
- Can you manage the financial commitment of ongoing treatment?

One often overlooked aspect of candidacy is timing. Life circumstances can significantly impact treatment success. During my assessment, I realized that starting treatment just before a major work project wouldn't set me up for success. Instead, I chose to begin when I could fully focus on establishing new routines and managing potential side effects.

Your healthcare provider will also want to understand your weight loss history and previous attempts at weight management. This information helps determine if medication is appropriate and which type might work best for you. Be prepared to discuss:

- Previous weight loss attempts and outcomes
- Patterns of weight gain and loss
- Specific challenges that have hindered success
- Current eating habits and exercise routines
- Stress levels and sleep patterns

The assessment process should feel collaborative rather than judgmental. When I shared my frustration about regaining weight after previous diets, my healthcare provider explained how this pattern actually supported my candidacy for medication, as it demonstrated the need for additional tools beyond willpower alone.

It's essential to approach the assessment process with complete honesty - both with your healthcare provider and yourself. Medications work best when prescribed to appropriate candidates who are ready to fully engage with treatment. Remember, being deemed not ready or suitable for medication isn't a personal failure - it's about finding the right tool for your specific situation at the right time.

If you're considering weight loss medication, start by scheduling a comprehensive consultation with a healthcare provider who specializes in weight management. Prepare for this appointment by:

- Gathering your complete medical history
- Documenting your weight loss attempts and outcomes
- Listing all current medications and supplements
- Recording your typical eating and exercise patterns
- Writing down specific questions about treatment

This thorough evaluation process might seem daunting, but it's designed to ensure your safety and maximize your chances of success. Through my own journey, I've learned that understanding and meeting these criteria isn't about qualifying or failing - it's about finding the most appropriate path to sustainable weight management for your unique situation.

Lifestyle Readiness: Evaluating Your Commitment to Long-Term Success

Starting weight loss medication represents a significant commitment that extends far beyond simply taking a pill each day. Success requires lifestyle readiness - a state of mental, emotional, and practical preparation that positions you for sustainable results. Through my journey with Zepbound, I've learned that the medication serves as a powerful tool, but your lifestyle readiness determines how effectively you can use that tool.

One evening, while organizing my weekly medication and meal planning routine, I reflected on how different my approach to weight management had become. The structured nature of medical weight loss required me to develop new systems and habits that I hadn't previously considered necessary. This realization highlighted how lifestyle readiness isn't just about willingness - it's about creating sustainable structures that support long-term success.

Evaluating your lifestyle readiness involves honest assessment of your daily routines and habits. Consider how medication requirements will fit into your:

- Morning and evening routines
- Work schedule and commitments
- Social and family obligations
- Exercise and activity patterns
- Meal planning and preparation time

The commitment to weight loss medication extends beyond personal readiness to include your support network. During my journey, I discovered that having conversations with family members about my treatment plan wasn't optional - it was essential for creating an environment conducive to success. Their understanding and support made it easier to maintain new habits and navigate challenges.

To assess your lifestyle readiness, ask yourself these crucial questions:

- Can I commit to taking medication consistently at the prescribed times?
- Am I willing to modify my eating habits and food choices?
- Do I have the time for regular medical check-ups?
- Can I maintain detailed records of my progress and side effects?
- Am I prepared to handle potential social situations differently?

Practical preparation plays a vital role in lifestyle readiness. My success with weight loss medication began when I created systems to support my journey. I developed a medication tracking system, established regular meal prep routines, and reorganized my schedule to accommodate new habits. This foundation of practical support proved essential for maintaining consistency with treatment.

Lifestyle readiness also means being prepared for challenges and setbacks. During my first month on medication, an unexpected work trip tested my new routines. Having thought through such scenarios in advance helped me maintain my treatment plan despite the disruption. This experience taught me that lifestyle readiness includes developing contingency plans for various situations.

To evaluate your practical readiness, consider implementing these preparatory steps:

- Create a medication tracking system
- Establish regular meal planning routines
- Organize your schedule to accommodate new habits
- Develop strategies for challenging situations
- Set up a support network communication plan

Remember that lifestyle readiness isn't about perfection - it's about having the right mindset and systems in place to support your journey. When I began treatment, I wasn't perfectly prepared for every challenge, but I had developed enough structure and support to adapt and learn as I progressed.

Your commitment to lifestyle changes will evolve as you progress through treatment. Initially, focus on establishing basic routines and support systems. As you become more comfortable with the medication's effects, you can refine and adjust your approach based on what works best for you.

Being lifestyle-ready means understanding that weight loss medication is a tool to support your journey, not a magic solution. Success requires active engagement with the treatment process, consistent effort in maintaining new habits, and the flexibility to adapt as your needs change. By thoroughly evaluating your lifestyle readiness before beginning treatment, you set yourself up for sustainable success in your weight management journey.

The Consultation Checklist: Essential Questions for Your Healthcare Provider

Walking into your healthcare provider's office prepared with the right questions can make the difference between a productive consultation and a missed opportunity. During my first weight loss medication consultation, I wished I'd had a comprehensive list of questions ready. Now, after years of experience and countless conversations with other patients, I've developed a thorough checklist that ensures you get the most from your appointment.

At your consultation, consider asking these essential questions about your medical history and current health status:

- What specific health markers indicate I'm a good candidate for weight loss medication?
- How do my current medications interact with weight loss drugs?
- What health conditions might disqualify me from treatment?
- How will my age and hormonal status affect treatment options?
- What tests or screenings should I complete before starting medication?

The first time I met with my doctor about Zepbound, I was surprised by how much my complete medical history mattered. Even minor details about past medications and family health patterns helped shape my treatment plan. This experience taught me the importance of gathering comprehensive health information before the consultation.

Questions about the medication itself should include:

- Which specific medication do you recommend for my situation and why?

- What is the expected timeline for seeing results?
- How long will I need to take this medication?
- What are the most common side effects for this specific medication?
- How will we monitor my progress and adjust dosage if needed?

One afternoon, while reviewing my treatment plan with my healthcare provider, I realized how crucial it was to understand the practical aspects of medication management. This led me to develop additional questions about day-to-day medication use:

- What time of day should I take the medication?
- How should I handle missed doses?
- What dietary restrictions come with this medication?
- How will the medication affect my exercise routine?
- What symptoms warrant immediate medical attention?

Financial and insurance considerations deserve careful attention during your consultation. Be sure to ask:

- Is this medication covered by my insurance?
- What are the out-of-pocket costs?
- Are there manufacturer discount programs available?
- How often will I need follow-up appointments?
- What additional costs should I anticipate for monitoring and testing?

The success of your weight loss journey often depends on understanding the support and resources available. Consider these questions about ongoing care:

- What support services do you offer for patients on weight loss medication?

- How often will we meet to monitor progress?
- What lifestyle changes should I implement alongside the medication?
- How can I prepare for potential challenges or plateaus?
- What resources do you recommend for additional support?

During my consultation, I found it helpful to take notes and bring a support person who could help remember important details. Consider recording the consultation (with permission) or asking for written materials about your treatment plan.

Prepare for your consultation by:

- Writing down your questions in advance
- Bringing a complete list of current medications and supplements
- Having a record of your weight history and previous weight loss attempts
- Preparing a typical daily food and activity log
- Bringing your insurance information and coverage details

Remember that no question is too basic or unimportant when it comes to your health. Your healthcare provider should welcome your questions and provide clear, understandable answers. If you don't understand something, ask for clarification.

After your consultation, schedule any recommended tests promptly and begin gathering the resources you'll need for successful treatment. Create a system for tracking questions that arise between appointments, and don't hesitate to contact your healthcare provider's office if urgent concerns develop.

The consultation process is your opportunity to build a strong foundation for successful weight loss treatment. By coming prepared with these questions, you demonstrate your commitment to the process and ensure you have the information needed to make informed decisions about your health journey.The decision to start weight loss medication represents a pivotal moment in your health journey - one that deserves careful consideration and thorough preparation. Throughout this chapter, we've explored the essential elements that contribute to making an informed choice about weight loss medication, from medical criteria to lifestyle readiness and crucial consultation questions.

As a reminder, your readiness for weight loss medication depends on several key factors that we've discussed:

- Medical eligibility and health status
- Lifestyle preparedness and support systems
- Financial and practical considerations
- Personal commitment to long-term changes
- Understanding of medication benefits and risks

As you consider whether weight loss medication is right for you, remember that this decision isn't about meeting an arbitrary standard - it's about finding the most appropriate tool for your unique health journey. The thoroughness of your preparation will significantly impact your potential for success. The tools and insights provided in this chapter can help guide you toward making an informed decision that aligns with your health goals and personal circumstances.

Whether you decide that weight loss medication is right for you now, later, or not at all, the evaluation process itself offers valuable insights into your health journey. Use this knowledge to make a decision that feels right for your unique situation, knowing that you've considered all the essential factors.

As we move forward into exploring how to integrate medications with lifestyle changes in the next chapter, carry forward the understanding that successful weight management is a comprehensive journey that combines medical intervention with personal dedication and lifestyle modification. Your thoughtful consideration of whether weight loss medication is right for you sets the foundation for whatever path you choose to pursue.

INTERVIEWS WITH GLP-1 USERS

Interview with Julie

Interview with Julie: The Journey of Losing 150 Pounds and Finding Balance

Q1: Julie, take us back to the moment you decided to make a change. What was your breaking point?

Julie:

I wish I could say it was some grand, life-altering revelation, but honestly? It was just me, sitting on my couch, out of breath after tying my shoes. That moment hit hard. I was 300 pounds, exhausted all the time, and every doctor I saw had a new warning about my health. But the real kicker? I didn't recognize myself anymore.

I wasn't just physically heavy—I was carrying around this weight of unhappiness. Every day felt like I was waiting for something to magically fix itself. But then I realized... no one was coming to save me. If I wanted to change, I had to create it.

Q2: What made you choose a GLP-1 drug, and how did it impact your journey?

Julie:

I had tried everything. Diets, extreme workouts, fasting—if there was a trending weight-loss hack, I had done it. Nothing worked long-term because I had a fundamental issue with hunger and control.

A doctor mentioned GLP-1 medications to me, and at first, I was skeptical. A shot to help me lose weight? It sounded too good to be true.

But after doing my research, I realized this wasn't just about appetite suppression—it was about resetting my relationship with food.

The first few weeks were rough (the side effects can make you rethink your choice), but then something amazing happened—I wasn't thinking about food every second of the day. The "food noise" in my head disappeared. For the first time, I could make intentional choices instead of feeling like I was at war with my own cravings.

Q3: You mentioned switching to an off-market Tirzepatide. Why did you make that decision?

Julie:

Oh, the classic insurance denial saga—fun times.

After my initial success on a GLP-1 drug, my insurance decided I was no longer "qualified" because I had lost weight. Insurance can be crazy and difficult sometimes. The cost out-of-pocket was astronomical, and I wasn't about to drop \$1,000+ a month just to maintain my progress.

That's when I started looking into online providers and compounding pharmacies. I found a reputable source and switched to an off-market version of Tirzepatide. It worked exactly the same. And honestly? If I had waited around for the system to help me, I'd probably be back where I started. Sometimes, you have to take control of your own health—ethically, of course, but also realistically. Thankfully, there are options these days outside of insurance.

Q4: You've lost 150 pounds. That's an incredible achievement! But what's been the hardest part of keeping it off?

Julie:

Oh boy. Where do I start?

Losing the weight was physical. Keeping it off is mental.

I still struggle with what I call "fat girl brain." Even at my healthiest, I sometimes catch myself thinking like I'm still 300 pounds—avoiding chairs with armrests, hesitating to walk upstairs in front of people (because old me would have been gasping for air), or feeling like I don't deserve to wear a certain outfit.

And let's talk about food guilt. Undoing that wiring isn't easy when you've spent decades equating food with comfort. Sometimes, I'll have a piece of cake, and suddenly, my brain whispers, Well, you've ruined everything. Might as well eat the whole thing.

That's where the occasional use of Tirzepatide helps me. If I notice old habits creeping back—overeating or snacking mindlessly—I use it as a tool to reset, not as a crutch. I never want to rely on it completely, but it's like having a safety net when my discipline wavers.

Q5: A lot of people assume losing weight automatically makes you happy. Has that been your experience?

Julie:

Yes and no.

Am I happier now? Absolutely. My body moves more easily, I feel more confident, and my health markers are so much better. But did losing weight magically fix all my problems? Nope.

I still have insecurities. I still have bad days. I still get emotional and think, Screw it, I deserve fries and a milkshake.

What changed was my ability to course-correct. I have a sense of control now. Before, food controlled me. Now, I control it. And that freedom? That's what makes me truly happy.

Q6: What advice would you give to someone considering GLP-1 medications or starting a major weight loss journey?

Julie:

Oh, I have so many things to say. But let me give you my top five takeaways:

1. This isn't a magic fix. The meds help, but you still have to do the work—changing habits, moving your body, and making better choices.
2. Ignore the haters. People will have opinions, especially about GLP-1 drugs. Some will say it's cheating, and others will judge your methods. Ignore them. Your journey is yours alone.
3. Be patient with your brain. Your body will change faster than your mindset. Give yourself grace as you adjust to your new normal.
4. Plan for maintenance. Weight loss is one phase—keeping it off is another battle entirely. Have a strategy for long-term success, whether it's continued medication, lifestyle changes, or a mix of both.
5. You are more than a number. The scale doesn't define you. Don't tie your worth to your weight. Ever.

Q7: Final question—what's one thing you wish people understood about weight loss and GLP-1 drugs?

Julie:

That it's not about being skinny—it's about being free.

Free from food obsession. Free from health issues. Free from feeling like your body is holding you hostage.

This journey isn't about looking good in a bikini (though, hey, that's a nice perk). It's about reclaiming your life. And if a medication can help someone do that, why should there be shame in using it? I will add that the emotional work is ongoing, as with anyone (thin or heavy), but I have tackled one of my stumbling blocks, and I am physically healthier and ready to tackle other parts of my life.

If I could go back and talk to 300-pound me, I'd tell her:

"You're not broken. You're not weak. You just need the right tools to help you. And once you have them? You're unstoppable."

Interview with Jeff: Turning His Health Around at 65

Q1: Jeff, tell us about the moment you realized you needed to change. What was your wake-up call?

Jeff:

Oh, there were plenty of warning signs—my doctor had been waving the red flag for years—but the moment it really hit me? I was sitting in his office, looking at my bloodwork, and he said, "Jeff, if you don't make some serious changes, you're heading toward a heart attack, stroke, or worse."

That scared me. I had always told myself, I'll get around to losing the weight someday, but someday kept getting pushed further away. Meanwhile, my knees were shot, my blood sugar was through the roof, and my cholesterol levels were a disaster. And still, I was eating and drinking like I was invincible.

That day, I realized: I'm running out of somedays.

Q2: You tried Monjouro for 18 months. How did you decide on this medication, and what was it like in the beginning?

Jeff:

I'll be honest—at first, I thought it was just another gimmick. I'd tried diets before, lost a few pounds, and always gained it back. But my doctor explained that Monjouro wasn't just about weight loss—it was about getting my diabetes under control and retraining my brain around food. That part intrigued me.

The first few weeks? Rough. My appetite tanked, and I felt like I had the flu. But then, something amazing happened—I stopped obsessing over food. The cravings that had ruled my life for decades? They just… faded.

For the first time, I could eat because I was hungry, not because I was bored, stressed, or just wanted to indulge. That was a game-changer.

Q3: Losing 145 pounds is incredible. What were some of the biggest challenges along the way?

Jeff:

Oh man, where do I start?

1. Breaking lifelong habits. I had built my life around food and drinks—weekends out, big meals, celebrating with food. It was a total mindset shift to find new ways to enjoy life that didn't revolve around eating.
2. Staying motivated. The weight came off fast at first, but after the initial big drop, it slowed down. I had to remind myself that progress is progress—even if it's just a pound here or there.
3. Dealing with social situations. People don't realize how much of our lives revolve around food. Saying "no" to second helpings, cutting back on alcohol—it was an adjustment, and some friends didn't get it.
4. The physical changes. Losing weight was great, but after years of carrying 320 pounds, my knees were still paying the price. I had to strengthen my muscles and be patient with my body as it adjusted.

Q4: You're now tapering off Monjouro. How do you feel about maintaining your progress?

Jeff:

Terrified. But also hopeful.

This medication gave me the kickstart I needed, but now it's up to me to keep doing the work. I'm still meal planning, still tracking my weight, still hitting the gym. The difference is, I don't feel out of control anymore.

I'm also in a totally different place mentally. Before, if I had a bad day, I'd spiral—one bad meal would turn into a bad week, then a bad month. Now? If I slip up, I just get right back on track. No guilt, no shame—just forward motion.

Q5: You mentioned keeping up with your wife—how has your weight loss changed your lifestyle?

Jeff:

My wife has always been the active one. She's been hiking, biking, doing yoga—and I was always the guy saying, "You go ahead, I'll meet you at the bar."

Now? We're doing it together. We take long walks, travel, try new things—because I can. I'm not sidelined by my weight anymore. I never want to go back to watching life from the sidelines.

Q6: If you could go back and talk to your 320-pound self, what would you say?

Jeff:

I'd grab myself by the shoulders and say:

"You're stronger than you think. You don't have to live this way. The food, the drinks, the lifestyle—it's not worth what you're losing in return."

Because that's what I didn't see at the time—I was losing so much. Not just my health, but my ability to fully live my life.

Q7: What advice would you give to someone who feels stuck in their weight loss journey?

Jeff:

1. Find your 'why.' I had to get real with myself—if I didn't change, my future was bleak. Find the thing that drives you and hold onto it.
2. Be patient. You didn't gain the weight overnight, and you won't lose it overnight either. Trust the process.
3. Use every tool available. Medication, therapy, support groups—there's no shame in getting help. Do what works for you.
4. Don't go it alone. Having support—whether from family, friends, or a community—makes a huge difference.
5. Forgive yourself and keep going. There will be setbacks. That doesn't mean you've failed. Just keep moving forward.

Q8: Final thoughts—what's life like for you now, at 175 pounds?

Jeff:

It's like I've been given a second shot at life.

I'm healthier, stronger, and more active than I've been in decades. My knees don't scream at me when I walk. My doctor barely recognizes me. My bloodwork? Perfect.

But more than that—I just feel good. I wake up with energy. I move with ease. I'm not thinking about my weight all day, every day. I'm just living. And that's the biggest win of all.

Interview with Maria (47, wants to lose 20 lbs. quickly)

Avery: Maria, thanks so much for sitting down with me today. Can you share a bit about why you decided to try GLP-1 medications?

Maria: Glad to talk with you, Avery. Honestly, it started with my daughter's wedding approaching. I've been feeling intense pressure to drop around 20 pounds quickly. Living in LA, you know how it is—there's this unspoken expectation to always look perfect, especially for something as big as your child's wedding.

Avery: Have you always felt this way about your body?

Maria: Looking back, I realize I've always been pretty hard on myself. In my younger days, especially in college, I could eat literally anything without worrying. But after turning 40, my body changed. Suddenly, I had to think twice about everything I ate. Truthfully, my weight isn't medically problematic—I'm actually pretty healthy overall—but because of family health issues, and probably a bit of body-image pressure from being in LA, I've convinced myself I needed to drop those extra pounds. I admit, I might have been chasing a bit of an unrealistic ideal.

Avery: So how did GLP-1 meds come into the picture?

Maria: My girlfriends talked about it constantly, claiming it was this miracle solution to shed weight quickly. I jumped on board without giving it much thought, definitely not realizing it was something I should discuss seriously with a doctor first.

Avery: What was your experience like starting the medication?

Maria: Honestly, it was pretty rough right away. Severe nausea, terrible stomach pain, and exhaustion hit me almost immediately. There was one particularly bad evening—I missed my daughter's dress fitting because I felt too sick to leave the couch. That was when I realized I'd underestimated how serious this could be. Honestly, I felt embarrassed and annoyed that I had trusted my friend's casual recommendation without doing my own homework.

Avery: Did you seek medical help at that point?

Maria: Not initially, unfortunately. I bought the medication online based purely on my friend's recommendation without checking with a healthcare professional first. Eventually, though, the side effects got so intense I finally reached out to my doctor, who helped me realize how important professional guidance really is.

Avery: It sounds like that was a big turning point. What did you do next?

Maria: I decided to stop taking the medication entirely and regrouped. I focused on finding healthier, more balanced ways to approach weight loss and overall well-being, both physically and emotionally. It was a big relief to shift toward something sustainable rather than chasing unrealistic shortcuts.

Avery: What's your advice to others considering GLP-1 medications?

Maria: Do not rush it. Educate yourself thoroughly, speak with your doctor, and consider if it's even right for your situation. Your health is far more important than quickly dropping a few pounds for an event.

Avery: How are you feeling about everything now?

Maria: I'm feeling better and more grounded. Honestly, it was an important wake-up call for me to prioritize long-term health over quick fixes. I still want to feel great at my daughter's wedding, but now I understand that truly feeling good is about more than just looking good in a dress.

Avery: Thanks for being so candid, Maria. Your honesty will really resonate with others.

Maria: Thank you, Avery. It feels good to talk about it openly—I hope it helps someone avoid my mistakes.

Interview with David (27, 6', 265 lbs)

Avery: David, it's awesome to have you here today. Tell us a bit about what led you to try GLP-1 medications for weight loss.

David: Glad to be here, Avery. Honestly, it hit me after a recent doctor's appointment. At 27, hearing my blood work was showing some early signs of trouble really shook me. My family tree isn't doing me any favors—heart disease on my dad's side, diabetes on my mom's. Plus, I realized pretty quickly after college that my body was not handling the "eat whatever I want" diet anymore. I used to be able to eat pizza at midnight without a second thought, but suddenly my body was like, "Hey, maybe not!" It became clear that I needed something more than just salads and occasional workouts to tackle this.

Avery: Have you always had a hard time losing weight?

David: Pretty much, yeah. But things got way tougher about two years ago when I started anti-anxiety meds. Don't get me wrong, they really helped me manage my anxiety, but suddenly, I found myself gaining weight even though I wasn't changing much about my lifestyle. Losing that extra weight felt impossible, like trying to climb a slippery slope.

Avery: That's so relatable for many people. What made GLP-1 specifically appealing to you?

David: My doctor and I talked through a bunch of options, and GLP-1 came up because it directly targets appetite and helps manage blood sugar. Given my family history and medication-related challenges, it felt like exactly what I needed to regain control.

Avery: Your regular doctor couldn't prescribe it directly, right? How did you navigate that?

David: Right. That was tricky. I did tons of research, joined a few online groups, and eventually found a reliable Telehealth service that could prescribe it remotely. It wasn't cheap since insurance didn't cover it, but my wife and I decided the investment in my health was worth it.

Avery: How was your experience when you first started the medication? Any side effects?

David: Honestly, The first couple of weeks were a bit rough. I had some nausea and felt pretty tired. After four weeks, my provider increased my dose, and I'll be real—there was about a week of serious stomach upset and nausea. I even joked with my wife, "Is this what pregnancy morning sickness feels like?" Thankfully, that passed, and now things are feeling much better.

Avery: Glad to hear that. Have you had any encouraging successes since you started?

David: Yeah, it's actually been pretty motivating. I've dropped around 10 pounds in just over a month, and more importantly, I'm finally feeling energized again. The best part? One day, I woke up and realized I'd actually forgotten about snacking—I didn't even crave my usual midnight raid on the pantry.

Avery: That's fantastic progress! Have you thought much about your long-term plans with GLP-1?

David: I have, and ideally, I'd like to use this medication as a stepping stone toward healthier habits. I'd love to reach a point where I might not need it anymore, but honestly, I'm open to sticking with it if that's what keeps me healthy. It's all about seeing how my body responds long-term.

Avery: Are you making sure to keep your regular doctor and your Telehealth provider updated?

David: Totally. I know it's crucial. My GP and the Telehealth doc both have my full health picture—every detail, from my weight changes to side effects and blood tests. It's important to catch anything unusual early and make sure I'm staying safe while making progress.

Avery: Have you shared with others that you're taking this medication?

David: Honestly, no. My wife is the only one who knows. There's still stigma around medications for weight loss and mental health, so I've kept it private. It just feels easier that way.

Avery: Has that privacy made getting the support you need harder?

David: Maybe a bit, but luckily, my wife is amazing and supportive. I am considering joining some online communities or working with a health coach—somewhere I can talk openly without worrying about judgment.

Avery: Great insight. What's your ultimate goal with this journey?

David: My goal is pretty simple—I want to feel healthy and vibrant again. I want to be able to fully enjoy my marriage, grow my business, and eventually start a family. It'd also be nice to go hiking or run around with our dog without getting winded halfway through.

Avery: Those goals are fantastic, David. Thanks so much for being open and real about your experiences. I'm sure many readers will connect with your story.

David: Thank you, Avery. It feels good to talk about this openly.

AVERY'S PERSONAL 16 WEEK TIRZEPATIDE JOURNAL

The Unexpected Road to Health and Happiness...

Right as the pandemic turned our lives upside down, I got a job offer that took me from Boston all the way across the country to sunny Los Angeles. For reasons that are far too predictable to bore you with, I packed up my life and embraced the adventure.

If you've never been to California, the best way I can describe it is "Paradise with a Price Tag." The weather is nearly perfect, the people are endlessly fascinating (and fun to gossip about), shopping is incredible, and there's always something beautiful to see or inspiring to do. But paradise isn't free—living here can drain your wallet pretty quickly. For me, there was another cost, too: being separated from my family and friends by an entire country during the isolation of the pandemic.

I share this so you can understand the backdrop of my journey. Moving to California was amazing and transformative at that point in my life. The pandemic? Not so much—but we've all written and read enough blogs about that, so let's skip ahead.

My true journey toward health and longevity started in California, and let me tell you, I was late to the party—I was already in my 50s! But better late than never, right? I dove headfirst into California's outdoor lifestyle, enjoyed the endless healthy food options, and even explored the "woo woo" culture. Yes, I mean manifestation, crystals, astrology, meditation, and taking mental health seriously.

It didn't take long for me to realize that I hadn't been living authentically (to borrow a very Californian phrase) for the past 25+ years. One of my biggest revelations was that I wanted to maximize the time I have left on this earth, living fully and authentically. It was time to get my body and mind in sync with my new outlook.

After soaking up every bit of fun and freedom LA had to offer, I decided it was time to head back east. But California had spoiled me, and I knew I couldn't handle another Boston winter. Instead, I opted for Florida, giving myself six months to figure out my next move.

Florida became my personal retreat. I walked four miles every day, ditched alcohol and sugar, swapped nightly TV for meditation, and truly focused on my goals. It was fantastic, but let's be real—it wasn't sustainable in the long term. I'm not independently wealthy, nor am I someone who thrives on endless planning. I'm an idea and action person at heart.

Even though the extreme regimen didn't last, I noticed positive changes in my body and mindset. There was a catch, though—family history. My dad had Type 2 Diabetes, high cholesterol, and high blood pressure. My mom battled dementia, high cholesterol, and high blood pressure. Sadly, I lost them both within the last three years. The weight of their health struggles (literally and figuratively) made my own journey feel even more urgent.

Just as I was grappling with this uphill battle against genetics and a lifetime of unhealthy habits, something unexpected and wonderful happened—I fell in love!

Love Is Fattening

I fell in love! It's amazing and transformative in so many ways. Sharing your life with someone who excites you, challenges you, and makes everything more fun was exactly what I'd dreamed of—and precisely what was on my manifestation list.

As a gay woman in my 50s, the dating pool felt simultaneously too large and too small. There were plenty of first dates, fewer second ones, and even fewer beyond that. Nothing seemed to click. I even revisited dating men just to be sure... but nope, definitely not for me.

Then, miraculously, we matched on Hinge and immediately hit it off. Of course, there were hurdles. She was living in Miami, while I had just decided to move to New Orleans. This meant lots of weekend visits and remote working sessions to squeeze in more time together.

I share all of this to explain my "happiness weight gain." You know the type—when you meet someone wonderful and suddenly there are new restaurants to try, cocktails to sip, and lazy days spent lounging around, getting to know each other.

One year later, settled in New Orleans—a city famous for its irresistible cuisine—I found myself regaining the pounds I'd worked so hard to lose. Falling in love and enjoying life turned out to be deliciously fattening. Don't get me wrong; finding your person is rare and wonderful, like discovering a needle in a haystack, and I wouldn't trade my happiness for anything.

Still, I was faced with a new challenge: how to stay healthy while genuinely enjoying life—or even better, living my absolute best life. Was it possible to have both?

I decided to tackle the issue head-on. I'd been a fan of Dr. Mark Hyman's podcast, so when he introduced his Functional Health program—a comprehensive, affordable blood and urine test—I decided to give it a shot. At $500, including a six-month follow-up, it felt reasonable given the typical cost of healthcare.

Unsurprisingly, my test results were mixed. Some areas showed excellent health, but others, not so much. My weight had clearly become an issue again, and it was affecting my blood pressure, cholesterol levels, and blood sugar—all of which were elevated.

I quickly launched "Operation Healthy Living"…again. Unfortunately for me (but wonderfully for her), my partner is one of those lucky people who can eat steak, drink cocktails, snack on jellybeans before bed, and still have perfect test results. I love that for her—but I'm also a little jealous!

Reluctantly, I started blood pressure medication but stubbornly decided to tackle cholesterol through diet and lifestyle changes. However, progress was slow after a few months in New Orleans, my daughter's wedding, and a fabulous trip to Paris. My health markers improved slightly, but not enough. Balancing life's pleasures, especially post-menopause, work, and life responsibilities, made it challenging to focus exclusively on wellness.

Frustrated and nearing my wit's end, I entered what I now affectionately call the "Tirzepatide Times."

Tirzepatide Times: Week One – Welcome to the BLEK Zone

I chose to kick off my Zepbound adventure on a Sunday. Why Sunday, you ask? Because I thought it sounded like a responsible adult move—post-Paris trip but pre-holiday madness. What could go wrong, right?

First, I was so unprepared that I had to YouTube how to give myself the injection. (Thank you, kind strangers on the internet) After a brief tutorial, I summoned my courage, gave myself the shot, and waited for something magical to happen……And waited.

By hour 36, I felt... weird. Not exactly sick, but not my normal fabulous self either. Weird morphed into the unholy trifecta of nausea, joint aches, and a headache that felt like thunder rumbling under my skull.

BLEK: The First Week Mood

The first week was a blur of BLEK, which, for the uninitiated, is a delightful combo of nausea and regret. It reminded me of the "morning sickness" era of my life. (Note to self: listen when smart people talk). Turns out, those pesky side effects everyone warns you about. They aren't kidding.

If I could turn back time, I would've taken my doctor's advice and gotten nausea meds beforehand. Rookie mistake. But I rallied and reached out to my Tirzepatide squad (a.k.a. friends who are one year into this joyride) for advice. They generously shared their wisdom again…not to mention that they had already told me all of this before:

Drink water. Like, become a human aquarium.

Protein is your BFF. Chicken, fish, eggs, yogurt if you're fancy, bone broth.

Small bites = big energy. Grazing is the new dining.

Avoid junk food. Yes, we all know this, but now it's non-negotiable. That stuff'll kill you…literally.

Chill out. That first week is not for heroics; it's for naps.

Fun with Side Effects

Let me tell you, hydration is a full-time job on this medication. I'm not a water enthusiast on my best day, but the ahem, constipation situation made me a believer. A good mix of water and veggies worked wonders for my sluggish gut. Pre- and probiotics were like bringing a butter knife to a sword fight. I will admit to resorting to MiraLAX when things go really dry and ugly!

Protein cravings hit me hard. When chicken or fish felt like too much, I turned to bone broth. Who knew sipping savory liquid could feel so bougie? Pro tip: skip the sugary holiday drinks and grab some high-quality bone broth. It's like a warm hug for your stomach.

Small bites became my saving grace. I'm talking tiny bites every couple of hours. It's like grazing for survival. And honestly? It works.

Food Noise, Begone!

One friend nailed it when she said, "This shot turns off the food noise in my head." At first, I didn't get it. But by day seven, I realized I wasn't obsessing over snacks or fantasizing about dessert. I was eating because I needed to, not because I was bored or craving junk.

Week One Recap: Flu Vibes, But Worth It

By the end of week one, I was five pounds lighter. Sure, I felt like I'd had the stomach flu for a week, but hey, progress is progress. I may have been tired, but I was also determined to keep going. This is just the beginning of my Tirzepatide Times journey—stay tuned for weirder, wild, and hopefully less BLEK-filled updates!

Tirzepatide Times: Week Two – Lessons in Carbs, Cocktails, and Constipation

Week two kicked off in slow motion—sluggish, tired, and nauseous. Fatigue decided to unpack its bags and stay for a few days. I stuck to my small-bites strategy like a champ, but let's be real: when you feel like a human couch cushion, comfort food is your brain's natural SOS signal.

In theory, I should've doubled down on healthy choices (Kettle Bone Broth and Avocados work in a pinch). In reality? My cravings whispered sweet nothings about burgers and mashed potatoes. (Why do carbs always sound like the hero in these moments?) Even though I only had a couple of bites here and there, I knew I was caving.

When I did manage to coax myself into eating something green—hello, salad with tuna (arugula specifically fits the bill, and even canned salmon if I am out of tuna)—I felt like a whole new person. It's like my body said, "Finally, some respect!" That's when I realized this journey isn't just physical; it's a mental game, too. My comfort-food cravings weren't about hunger—they were my brain throwing a pity party and inviting all the bad decisions.

Weird Food Noise, Round Two

By day three, the fog started lifting. Suddenly, I wanted healthy food again. I even wanted more food—larger portions instead of nibbling like a squirrel all day. With more food came more energy, and just like that, life was looking up. I felt human again! Walking? Fun. Work? Manageable. Being social? Sure, why not!

Then came the curveball: I completely lost my desire to drink alcohol. Weird, right? Normally, I enjoy a glass of wine or a cocktail, especially living here in NOLA, where great food and drinks are practically a religion. But I wasn't feeling it even with a friend visiting for Thanksgiving weekend.

Of course, by Saturday, I was feeling so much better than I thought; why not have a couple of cocktails? I'll tell you why: the hangover from hell. Lesson learned. Tirzepatide and alcohol are not besties, and I will not be doing that again anytime soon. Sidebar: I have found that a glass of Vinho Verde goes down easily…but just one).

Week Two Wins (And Woes)

Despite my comfort food rebellion, Thanksgiving cocktails, and general sluggishness, I lost another three pounds! Cue happy dance. But more than that, I'm learning some valuable lessons about my relationship with food:

Quantity matters. (Duh, but still.)

Quality equals energy. (Also, duh, but apparently, I needed the reminder.)

My idea of "how much food I need" was way off.

I'm still marveling at how this tiny shot can change how I think about food. Somehow, the little wizardry in Tirzepatide is teaching me lessons I'd been ignoring for years. Even though I'm not a scientist, I'm planning to do some reading on blood sugar and weight loss—just to better understand what's happening. For the record, my blood sugar is in the normal range but on the higher side, so maybe this is a sign to dig deeper.

Quick Week Two Check-In

In case you're wondering, here's where I stand after week two:

Constipation? Still here, still a bummer.

Food budget? Thriving. I'm saving a ton on groceries and drinks.

Energy? Hit or miss, but improving.

Water intake? A struggle, but so necessary.

Seeing results? Super motivating!

Work in progress? Definitely—my food relationship is still under construction.

Week two taught me that this journey is about more than just weight loss. It's about breaking old habits, rewiring my brain, and figuring out what actually makes my body feel good. It's not easy, but it's worth it. The drug seems to be helping me manage this process – like a little support pet getting me over the finish line each week. Bring on week three!

Tirzepatide Times: Weeks Three & Four – Holidays, Hurdles, and a Little Letting Go

The holidays loomed like a beautifully decorated, sugar-coated landmine. Normally, I'm all in—the twinkling lights, the togetherness, the goodwill toward all, and, of course, the food and festive cocktails. But this year, I was eyeing the season with a mix of excitement and nervous energy.

Would I be too tired and sluggish to fully enjoy it? Would I be able to partake in the delicious holiday treats without feeling like I got hit by the Tirzepatide Truck?

Naturally, I did what any Type A, list-loving person would do—I made a plan:

Stick to the protein rule (eggs, fish, chicken, yogurt, almonds, bone broth, and yogurt). Stick with what I know.

Water, water, water. Stay hydrated or face the constipation consequences.

Sneak in veggies wherever possible. Think of it as a game. Spinach in eggs? Nailed it.

Balance morning walks with unapologetic afternoon naps. Because I am now a nap enthusiast.

Enjoy one or two bites of irresistible holiday sweets. (Read: five bites, but who's counting?)

Meditate daily to keep my Grinch tendencies at bay.

Journal my thoughts and worries. Because if I write them down, maybe they'll stop haunting me at 3 AM.

False Advertising & The Fitness Struggle

I got back to my walking and functional training routine, but let me tell you—motivated was not a word I would have used to describe myself. The commercials for Tirzepatide make it look like you'll be out here running a 10k, climbing mountains, and joyfully riding bikes into the sunset. Lies.

I thought maybe I was the problem (Am I lazy? Is this my new normal? Should I just accept that my couch and I are in a committed relationship?), so I reached out to others in the Zepbound Zone—turns out, I am not alone! Misery might not actually love company, but it sure is nice to know I'm not just imagining things.

The Mental Marathon

By week three, the fact that this wasn't just a physical journey—it was a full-on mental showdown- was hammered home yet again. I was losing weight, my clothes fit better, and I no longer felt bloated or heavy. But I wasn't quite at the point where people were complimenting me with that vague "Did you change your hair?" or "You look different!" comment.

And let's be real—the side effects were still a thing. Was it worth it? Some days, yes. Other days, I wondered if I was trading one set of problems for another.

Even with my well-intentioned holiday survival plan, I found it really hard to stick to it 100%. Week three felt like an internal tug-of-war between researching why I felt the way I did and just trusting my body to figure it out. The keyword of the week? Patience.

Week Four: Screw the List, Enjoy the Season

Somewhere between overthinking my protein intake and googling, "Why does Tirzepatide make me feel like a grandma on a long road trip?" I had an epiphany:

I needed to chill.

So, I did the unthinkable—I threw out the list and decided to just live my life. I let go of trying to micromanage every bite, every craving, every step.

Week four arrived, and with it, a blissful 10-day escape to Florida. The agenda? Walks by the water, relaxation, and soaking up time with friends and family.

I'd love to tell you that my diet magically improved, but come on—it was the holidays! Food temptations were everywhere, and instead of stressing about them, I decided to trust my gut (pun very much intended).

The best part? My body was finally adjusting to the medication. The nausea was fading, and I felt comfortable throughout the day for the first time. Progress!

Week Three & Four Takeaways:

Exercise motivation? Still MIA, but I'm working on it.

Food budgeting? Who knew I'd save so much by simply not wanting food…or cocktails?

Side effects? Easing up, thank goodness.

Water intake? Still my greatest challenge, but I'm doing my best.

Letting go of control? Surprisingly freeing.

Living my life? Yes. Finally.

Now, as I step into the new year, I'm realizing this journey is about more than weight loss—it's about redefining my relationship with not only food but also energy and my own expectations.

I'm not perfect, and this isn't a linear path, but I'm learning. And that, my friends, is something worth celebrating.

Tirzepatide Times: Week Five – Bliss, Blood Sugar, and a Break from the Crazy

If I had to sum up week five in one word, it would be **bliss**. I had a glimpse of this bliss during week four, but in week five, I'll take more of that. Thanks!

Yes, **bliss**. As in, side effects? Minimal. Energy? Back in action. Appetite? Oh, hey, there you are! It was like my body finally got the memo that we were doing this Tirzepatide thing long-term and decided to cooperate.

Don't get me wrong—I wasn't suddenly ravenous or daydreaming about devouring an entire pizza by myself. My appetite returned, but it was… normal. I ate when I was hungry, stopped when I was full, and somehow didn't need to mentally wrestle with myself over snacks. It felt like my relationship with food had gone from toxic ex to healthy friendship status.

The Scale: Slower, But Still Moving

I lost a pound a week during this stretch—not exactly headline-making results, but I'll take it. The slower pace didn't bother me as much as I expected. Maybe because I was too busy enjoying the perks:

My energy returned. I wasn't constantly thinking about when I could sneak in my next nap.

Protein remained my MVP. Chicken, eggs, fish, yogurt—if it packs a protein punch, I'm all in.

Sugar cravings? Yep, they made a few surprise appearances. I found myself wondering if my body was going through some weird sugar withdrawal. Was my blood sugar adjusting and making me miss the sweet stuff? Or was my inner cookie monster just trying to stage a comeback?

Whatever the cause, I stayed the course. When the cravings hit, I grabbed a protein-packed snack or, occasionally, gave in with a small treat—

because, let's be real, sometimes a bite of chocolate saves you from eating an entire cake later.

Alcohol: The Mystery of the Missing Desire

One weird but welcome change: my desire to drink alcohol completely vanished. As I have mentioned, I live in New Orleans—a place where laissez les bons temps rouler basically translates to "Would you like another cocktail?"—so this was surprising.

I can drink a glass of wine if I want to, and now it doesn't hit me like a freight train. But honestly? I just don't care about it anymore. It's like my body decided, We're good here. Hydrate or die-drate.

Don't get me wrong—when friends visit and we hit our favorite spots, I'll have a drink. And yep, I do get a little tipsy faster these days. (Cheap date alert!) But the appeal is gone. Maybe it's the blood sugar regulation. Or maybe Tirzepatide is my personal anti-wine fairy. Either way, my liver is probably throwing a party.

Decision Time: To Increase or Not to Increase

By the end of week five, I faced a decision: should I increase my dosage or stay the course? The typical move is to up the dose around this time, but I decided to hold off until week eight. My logic?

I feel good—like really good. Why mess with success?

I wanted to give my body time to fully settle into this new normal.

I actually needed to get some work done instead of napping through meetings.

I mean, if I can lose a pound a week without feeling like garbage, why rush into more side effects? Slow and steady seems to be working just fine.

The Unexpected Perks

It's not just about weight loss anymore. Sure, I'm happy my jeans aren't threatening to cut off my circulation, but other changes have caught my attention:

Blood pressure? Coming down! My doctor even mentioned we might talk about (gasp) lowering my dosage soon.

Cravings? Shifting toward healthier foods. I actually want a salad sometimes. Who am I?

Mindset? Clearer. I'm no longer hiding in the comfort-food bunker. I feel lighter—not just physically but mentally, too.

I'm genuinely looking forward to my bloodwork in February to see how my blood sugar and cholesterol levels have changed. For once, it feels like my health is on an upward trajectory instead of a constant battle. It is a relief to see change, feel change, and be in charge of change but still be able to go about my daily life. Let's face it: I am not a Hollywood starlet, and I do not get paid to keep myself trim and tight… and also menopause!

Gratitude, Grit, and the Cost of Health

While reflecting on these weeks, I couldn't help but think about how expensive these meds are for some people. I'm fortunate—my doctor prescribed it for health reasons, so I only pay $24 a month. (Yes, you read that right. Don't hate me.)

But knowing what I know now? I wouldn't put myself through those gnarly side effects just to fit into smaller jeans. My motivation was, and still is, my health. I needed to reset my metabolism, reduce my blood pressure, and avoid becoming best friends with insulin injections down the line.

The fact that I've lost weight along the way? Bonus.

Week Five Takeaways:

Protein is still king. Eggs, chicken, fish—my trifecta of success.

Water remains the MVP. Hydration is not optional if you want to avoid the constipation struggle.

Sugar cravings happen. But protein usually shuts them down.

Alcohol? Meh. My body's basically dry-curious without me even trying.

Patience pays off. Slow progress is still progress.

For the first time in a long time, I feel like my body and I are working together instead of battling for control. Here's to more good weeks ahead—minus the side effects and with plenty of protein-packed snacks.

Tirzepatide Times: Weeks 6, 7, & 8 – The Great Food Reunion & Temporary Amnesia

Weeks six through eight flew by in a happy blur of higher energy, zero constipation (hallelujah!), and food that actually tasted good again. I was eating with joy—real, genuine, oh-my-god-this-is-delicious joy.

You see, I have always loved food. Trying new restaurants? Yes, please. Sampling every dish at a tasting menu? Sign me up. Cooking at home like I'm auditioning for Top Chef? Used to be my thing. And for the first time in a long while, I felt like I was dipping my toe back into my normal life.

The numbers? Seventeen pounds down. Clothes fit better. Feeling lighter, both physically and mentally. I was winning.

And then… well, let's just say my inner food gremlin escaped its cage.

The "I Feel Great, Let's Eat Everything" Phenomenon

You know that feeling when you've been sick for ages, and the second you feel better, you suddenly need to make up for lost time? Like, I've been deprived long enough. Bring me ALL the things?

Yep. That was me. Despite my advanced wisdom, life experience, and the lessons I thought I had learned, I face-planted right into that trap.

And let me tell you… it was glorious.

I went out, ate the food, drank the drinks, and

enjoyed myself without overthinking every bite. It felt good.

Now, here's the kicker: I didn't lose any weight—but I didn't gain any either. That's when I realized something important…

So, Did I Forget Everything?

At first, it seemed like all my carefully learned habits had flown straight out the window like a rogue napkin on a windy day.

But here's the thing: I wasn't binging. I wasn't eating out of boredom, stress, or emotional turmoil. I was enjoying food again—on my terms.

And not gaining weight during this phase? That's a win. A few months ago, this kind of eating would have meant a guaranteed five-pound rebound. Now? My body seemed to be working with me instead of against me.

The Takeaways from My Little Food Reunion:

Food is fun again. And that makes me very happy.

My body knows what to do. No wild weight fluctuations = progress.

Balance is key. I may have temporarily ghosted my healthy habits, but I slid right back into my routine the second I stopped overindulging.

Seventeen pounds down feels really freaking good.

Now that I've had my moment of fun, I'm ready to rein things back in—not because I have to, but because I want to. My next goal? To find that perfect balance where I can enjoy my love of food without completely ignoring my progress.

Weeks 6, 7, & 8: A beautiful, delicious, weight-neutral blur. Bring on the next phase!

Tirzepatide Times: Weeks 9 & 10 – Big Girl Pants, Big Feelings, and a Big Dose of Reality

Weeks 9 and 10 brought a dose increase, a dose of dizziness, and a dose of deep thoughts—all served with a side of Mardi Gras madness.

I decided to put on my big girl pants (which, by the way, are now a size smaller—small wins!) and level up my Tirzepatide journey. But before making any changes, I had to check in with my doctor. This is standard practice with these meds—kind of like a progress report for grown-ups, except instead of grades, you get advice on side effects and an official green light to up the ante.

I felt great; my side effects were basically a thing of the past, and I was in a groove. So, when Dr. K casually said, "We should increase your dosage to 0.5 mL," I responded with an enthusiastic thumbs up!

Did I actually think through what that meant?

No. No, I did not.

Side Effects: The Sequel

Somewhere deep in my brain, I knew I should start mentally preparing for the side effect upgrade. But instead, I just blissfully carried on, convinced that I had somehow outgrown the nausea, exhaustion, and general BLEK.

Spoiler alert: I had not.

I gave myself the shot Monday morning, and by midday, I felt like a half-deflated balloon floating through life in a fog. Tired, nauseated, cranky—you name it. I was waiting (and waiting) to feel better.

And then came a fun, new side effect: dizziness. Not just a little lightheadedness—I'm talking full-on: why is the room tilting? kind of dizzy.

A quick call to my doctor led to some important revelations:

- Good news: My blood pressure had come down enough that we needed to adjust (aka lower) my meds. Big win!
- Not-so-good news: I had been slacking on water intake (whoops) and needed to drink a lot more. Turns out this can be a serious side effect so beware!
- Tough love news: I had to get my ass moving with some weight training to avoid losing muscle.

Ugh. Fine.

A Crucial Warning: Be Honest with Your Doctors!

I recently learned something important: If you are taking a weight loss medication, your doctors need to know—especially if you're having surgery or a medical procedure.

A friend of mine is having a colonoscopy, and she was told that it is critical to inform the anesthesiologist that she's on this medication. These drugs slow down digestion, meaning an "empty stomach" might not actually be empty—which can be life-threatening under anesthesia. This applies to any procedure, so if you're taking these meds, speak up!

This isn't just a Tirzepatide thing—it's a good reminder to always be honest with your healthcare providers about any meds you're taking. Advocating for yourself is a form of self-care. Be proactive and protect yourself!

The Weight Loss Mind Game

At this point, I had lost 20 pounds (yay!), my clothes fit better, and I could actually see the progress. So why didn't I feel more successful?

Despite the weight loss, something felt... off. Like I was caught in this strange in-between space where the results weren't dramatic enough to feel life-changing, but I also knew I was on the right path.

I realized my brain needed to catch up with my body.

Lesson learned: The mindset work on this journey is just as important as the physical changes. Weight loss isn't just about shedding pounds—it's about unlearning old habits, adjusting expectations, and getting comfortable in a changing body.

The "Taboo" Conversation

One unexpected side effect of this journey? People's reactions.

I've noticed that a lot of people taking weight loss meds don't like to admit it. There's a weird stigma attached—especially from those who have never been on them. I can immediately sense the shift if I casually mention it in conversation (only when relevant, of course).

Some people assume I must have Diabetes (which comes with its own set of opinions). Others act like I'm stealing a drug from those who 'really need it' (FYI: there is no shortage anymore). And then, of course, there are those who think I'm just taking the 'easy way out.'

Oh, and my personal favorite: "That's such a waste of money."

As it turns out, the cost per month is less than my coffee habit.

Here's the thing: I don't owe anyone an explanation. But I do find it interesting how polarizing this topic is. And let's be real—if someone had a magic pill for weight loss 20 years ago, we all know the line at the pharmacy would have been around the block.

Alcohol & Food: The Mardi Gras Challenge

I have almost completely given up alcohol, not because I'm forcing myself to, but because I just don't want it anymore.

Sure, if we go out to eat, I might have a glass of wine—but I barely finish it. Turns out, seltzer water with lime is my new best friend (who knew?). Bonus: skipping the extra cocktails helps balance out the times I go rogue with desserts or mashed potatoes.

Speaking of indulgences… Mardi Gras season is here.

If you live in New Orleans, you know this means party, party, party, and eat, eat, eat. And let's be honest, resisting holiday food was hard enough—Mardi Gras just took it up a notch.

But even with the side effects dragging me down, I still lost weight (which, considering the endless king cakes and fried everything around me, is basically a miracle).

Takeaways from Weeks 9 & 10:

- Side effects return when you increase your dose. Plan accordingly.
- Dizziness = a sign of real progress but also a signal to call your doctor! Lowering blood pressure meds? Huge milestone.
- Water is not optional. Skimping on hydration = instant regret.
- Weight training is necessary. (I hate that I just typed that.)
- Mental adjustments take time. My brain still needs to catch up with my progress.
- People have opinions. But they don't get to dictate my journey.
- Alcohol? Meh. Turns out I don't miss it.
- Mardi Gras + Tirzepatide = a true test of willpower.

See You on the Other Side (of Week 11!)

So here I am—20 pounds lighter, feeling better, thinking way too much about what this all means, and wondering what week 11 has in store for me.

Will I keep feeling better? Will my energy continue improving? Will I ever find the true motivation to lift weights? Stay tuned.

Tirzepatide Times: Weeks 11 & 12 – The Mind Games Begin

I'm not going to sugarcoat it—weeks 9 and 10 were a beast. Usually, I take my shot and have 36 hours of normalcy, and then BAM—hour 37 hits like a truck. Cue nausea, exhaustion, body aches, and occasional mood swings that could rival a dramatic movie monologue. Normally, it's manageable, but those two weeks? I felt stuck in a permanent state of BLEK.

Enter week 11, and hallelujah, I returned to my normally scheduled program. 🎉

Body vs. Brain: The Ultimate Showdown

I still have my 36-hour BLEK window, but at least now it's predictable. I know it will pass, and I'll feel like a functioning human again. What's fascinating, though, is how my hunger shifts throughout the week:

During the BLEK phase? No cravings. No thoughts of food. Just me, a couch, and my Kindle.

Post-BLEK? My appetite is back, and suddenly, I'm fantasizing about burgers, fries, and cookies.

My actual eating habits are much more mindful. I don't act on every craving, but I do acknowledge them and make conscious choices.

But here's the real surprise: I've started noticing mental shifts in other areas of my life, too.

The War on Old Habits

I've already mentioned how alcohol lost its appeal. That's still true. I might order a glass of wine out of habit, but half the time, I don't even want it. My body and brain seem to be on different pages, and it's weird.

But the biggest shocker? Shopping.

I used to love a good retail therapy session. Stress? Buy a cute top. Bored? Browse online for shoes I don't need. But lately, that urge has disappeared. I still shop when I need something, but that "I must buy all the things" energy? Gone.

Even grocery shopping has changed. I buy what I need, I get in, I get out. No more throwing in extra snacks or impulse buys. Part of me feels bad for my girlfriend—I never bring home anything fun anymore! But hey, at least we're saving money, right?

The Workout Hesitation (and a Pep Talk to Myself)

Since I'm finally feeling more like myself, I know it's time to ramp up my workouts. But confession: I feel nervous.

I know that my weight loss slows down when I start exercising more. That happened pre-Tirzepatide, too, so I shouldn't be surprised, but it still messes with my head.

Plus, I'll be honest—I feel out of shape. My body feels slightly weak, and stepping back into a real workout routine feels intimidating. But here's what I do know:

Strength training will help me keep my muscle while I lose fat.

I will feel better once I start.

The longer I wait, the more I'll psych myself out.

So, no more waiting. Time to get moving before my brain turns this into a bigger hurdle than it is.

Wardrobe Realities (AKA: The Eternal "I'll Fit Into This Someday" Closet)

I've lost 23 pounds now, and I'm tempted to run out and buy cute new clothes to celebrate. But I won't. Not yet.

Why? Because, like many women, I already own a whole mini department store of "someday" clothes. You know what I mean—those items we swore we'd fit into again, the ones with the tags still on them because they were a little too snug when we bought them.

So, for now, I'm shopping my own closet and celebrating the fact that my "too tight" section is slowly becoming my "fits just right" section.

My Current Survival Tactics

Hydrate beyond all reason. If I ever needed proof that drinking enough water matters, Tirzepatide delivered it.

Eat small bites often. This keeps the nausea at bay. I live by the "protein every couple of hours" rule now. I know, I know; I have said this every week, but it is worth repeating to you and myself!

Veggies are still hit or miss. I usually love veggies, but lately, I have to be strategic. The solution? Vegetable soup. On days when I feel 100%, I load up on salads and broccoli to make up for lost time.

Final Thoughts: Mindset is Everything

These past two weeks reminded me (for the 100th time) that weight loss is just as much a mental game as a physical one. My brain is still catching up to my new reality—whether it's food habits, exercise intimidation, or even shopping behavior.

But here's what I know for sure: I'm on the right track.

I may not be perfect, but I'm making progress. And honestly? That's all that matters.

See you in Week 13!

Tirzepatide Times: Week 13 – Blood Tests, Breakthroughs & a Birthday Win

I walked into **Week 13 with trepidation.** A while back, I scheduled my **follow-up blood tests with Function Health**, and, as time has a tendency to do, it **flew by faster than expected**. Suddenly, test day was staring me in the face.

And I *really* wanted to cancel.

You know that feeling when you *want* to know something, but at the same time, you're **afraid of what you might find out**? That was me.

Test Day Drama (Mostly in My Head)

The morning of the test, I **dragged myself to the lab**, caffeine-deprived and vitamin-free (*tragedy!*). These days, my **morning ritual** is practically sacred:

1. **AG1 first** – because I *swear* my life depends on it.
2. **Coffee.** Because, obviously.
3. **Protein-packed breakfast** – My go-to lately? **Seeduction toast with tzatziki, avocado, microgreens, and a poached egg.** Yes, it's **bougie**, and yes, eggs are basically a *luxury item* at this point, but hey—**it keeps me satisfied and crash-free.**

Instead of savoring my normal breakfast routine, I was **handing over blood and peeing in a cup.** Not quite as fun. But in **10 minutes, it was over**, and I could *finally* move on with my day.

By 3:00 PM? I was itching to see my results—because, wow, we are so used to instant information now, aren't we?

I logged in.

And there they were.

The Results Are In... And They're Amazing.

Every single one of my markers improved! 🎉

✅ **LDL (bad cholesterol):** Down **119 points**. *(What?! That's insane!)*

✅ **Glucose:** From **105 → 80.**

✅ **Kidney & liver function:** Back in **normal healthy ranges.**

✅ **A1C (which was already good):** From **5.5 → 5.0.**

Suddenly, all of those adjustments—the side effects, the weird cravings, the nausea—felt **100% worth it.**

At **22 pounds down** and with healthier blood markers, I was **feeling amazing** about my progress. And honestly? I think I had been *secretly* worried that my blood tests *wouldn't* show improvement.

It reminded me of something:

You know when you **buy a new hot water heater**? You *need* it, but it's not exciting. It's not **new furniture** or **beautiful curtains** you admire every day. It just *works*, and you take it for granted. But the moment you **get a hot shower**, you remember—**yep, that was a solid investment.**

That's how these test results felt. **Not flashy. Just essential.**

New Stress, New Symptoms?

Something I haven't mentioned in previous weeks: **I've noticed a weird new reaction to stress.**

Historically, stress for me has meant **headaches or sleepless nights**—never stomach issues. But lately? **If I feel suddenly stressed, my stomach is the first to react.**

This is **new territory** for me, and it's been a reminder to **actively manage stress**—whether through **meditation, deep breathing, or just stepping away from whatever is making me anxious.** It's fascinating how this journey isn't just about weight loss—it's about **understanding how my body is changing in ways I never expected.**

Other Wins from Week 13

- **The usual 36-hour adjustment period after my shot?** Still there, but **totally manageable** now that I *know* what to expect.
- **The constipation saga?** *Improving!* More **veggies + water = better days** all around.
- **My birthday happened!** 💐 And guess what? I went out, used my **birthday coupon at Anthropologie**, and bought **a dress I never would have fit into before.** That was **SO. MUCH. FUN.**

Final Thoughts: Progress You Can't Always See

This week reminded me that **progress isn't just about numbers on the scale**—it's also about **what's happening inside my body.**

Yes, I've lost weight. **But more importantly, I'm healthier.**

And *that* is what's going to **keep me moving forward.**

Onward to Week 14! 🚀

Tirzepatide Times: Week 14 – Travel, Compliments & Airport Hangovers

With **Mardi Gras season winding down** in New Orleans, we made the executive decision to skip the last rounds of parades and **trade beads for beach waves.** Five days of restful bliss in Florida? Yes, please.

First challenge: traveling with my **Tirzepatide shot cartridge** for the first time.

Let's be real—I'm **not a scientist** (😄), and I wasn't exactly thrilled about the idea of **letting my precious medication sit at room temperature for five days**. But, after re-reading the instructions (twice), **I trusted the process, and all was well.**

A Beach Break & The "You Look Amazing" Moment

Getting out of town was **exactly what I needed**—fresh fish, sandy toes, and a much-needed change of scenery. **We even made a quick stop in Miami for a day of fun with friends.**

And then, **it happened.**

The moment I had *kind of* been waiting for…

People I hadn't seen in months **noticed my weight loss** and said the magic words:

"Wow, you look amazing! What's your secret?"

I *wish* I could say I had some **inspirational, heartfelt response** prepared, but honestly? I went with **vague and breezy.**

I've learned that **mentioning GLP-1 meds** can sometimes bring *awkward silence* or unsolicited opinions, and I wasn't in the mood for that. **So, I accepted the compliments, thanked them, and moved on.**

Bathing Suits & Beach Confidence

Okay, let's talk about **the best part of this trip.**

My bathing suit fit better! 🎉

I felt **more comfortable on the beach** than I had in *ages*, which was a huge win.

But here's where I *disappointed myself* a little—I usually **love** my long waterfront walks in Florida, but this time? **I was kind of lazy.** I opted for maximum relaxation instead of my usual **power walks.**

Was it a mistake? No.

But do I want to be more active on my next trip? Absolutely.

Still, **one thing I did right**—I stuck to my **shot schedule**, taking it Monday morning before heading home on Tuesday (aka: before any side effects had time to crash my travel party).

Airport Food Struggles Are Real

Maneuvering **airport food options** is *always* a challenge.

Even when I **try** to make good choices, airport food is like:

✈️ **"Here's some sodium, sugar, and regret wrapped in plastic."**

By the time I land, **I'm either bloated, exhausted, or craving a salad like my life depends on it.** (Cue the **airport hangover.**)

What works for me?

✔️ **Water, water, and more water.** Yes, it means more bathroom breaks, but hydration is **worth it.**

✔️ **Veggies & hummus.** (Even if they aren't organic, *we survive.*)

✔️ **Greek yogurt.** Decent protein + easy to find.

✔️ **Fresh fruit** (*when it's not $10 for three grapes*).

What I avoid like a delayed flight:

🚫 Deli meats & cheeses (*always sketchy in an airport*).

🚫 Salty snacks & sweets (*instant regret*).

🚫 Alcohol (*Not that I drink anymore, but if I did? HARD PASS on drinking at altitude*).

I *wish* I was the kind of person who could **pack the perfect travel snack bag**, but **it just never happens.** So, that goes on the list of things to research and attempt next trip.

Coming Home & Finding My Routine Again

By the time we got back, **I wasn't sure if I was exhausted from the shot or just from travel itself.** (*Probably both.*)

I love **going away for a reset**, but nothing beats **coming home to my dogs and my own bed.**

This trip **made me realize something big:**

Routine is my friend. But at the same time, **I love traveling.**

So, the goal? **Find ways to keep a flexible routine** so I can **keep my energy up** while still **enjoying the adventure of new places.**

Week 14 Takeaways:

✔️ **Traveling with Tirzepatide?** ☑️ Easier than expected.

✔️ **Seeing results & getting compliments?** ☑️ Feels amazing.

✔️ **More beach confidence?** ☑️ Huge win.

✔️ **Airport food still sucks?** ☑️ No surprise there.

✔️ **Finding a balance between routine & adventure?** 🤔 Still a work in progress.

I almost forgot, down 22 pounds!

Tirzepatide Times: Week 15 – Reflection, Gratitude & The Making of a New Me

This week has been about **reflection and gratitude**.

I've been working a lot lately, and for me, work always comes with **a side of deep thinking**—about my business, about success, about what really matters. **This week, I decided to apply that same energy to my health journey.**

It's funny how we spend so much time defining **what success looks like in work, in relationships, in financial goals**—but how often do we stop to ask, *What does success in my health actually look like?*

So, I did what any deep-thinking, slightly over-caffeinated person would do: **I called my friend Emily.**

Conversations That Change Perspectives

Emily and I have a lot in common—including the fact that we're both on a **GLP-1 medication**. Our conversation this week wasn't about **side effects or meal plans**—it was about something much bigger:

The mental shift that happens when you stop just "getting through" the weight loss process and start actually thinking about what comes next.

At **25 pounds down**, I feel like I've hit both a **physical and mental milestone**.

Yes, my body is changing—**my clothes fit better, I'm not bloated, and I don't feel the need to suck in my stomach every five minutes.** But what's even more interesting?

I feel **more confident**—in small, everyday ways. Not just in how I look, but in how I carry myself. **Like my body is no longer something I have to manage or hide—it just *is*. And that's a big deal.**

Breaking the "More Than I Need" Habit

One of the biggest adjustments I'm still working on?

Unlearning the habit of expecting to be hungrier than I actually am.

For decades, my brain has been wired to **assume I'll want more food than I really need.** It's a strange feeling to sit down for a meal, get excited about something delicious, and then realize that **three bites in—I'm actually satisfied.**

I *can* still eat the foods I love, but I don't *need* as much as my mind is used to expecting.

Does that even make sense? It's like my stomach is writing a whole new script, and my brain is still flipping through the old pages, trying to catch up.

The Great Mystery: Why Did I Lose My Taste for Alcohol But Not Sweets?

Remember when I mentioned that **alcohol no longer appeals to me?** Still true. I'll have a glass of wine occasionally, but even when I do, it's more out of **habit** than actual desire.

But sweets? **Sweets still call my name.**

Why alcohol and not sugar? **Wouldn't they be in the same "craving" category?** Apparently not.

The good news? **A bite or two is enough now.** I don't have the **overwhelming need** to devour the entire dessert—just a taste satisfies me. And honestly, that feels like a win.

Shifting from "Survival Mode" to "Long-Term Success"

This week, I asked myself something I *should* have thought about earlier:

👉 **What does long-term success in my health actually look like?**

- How do I maintain **my improved blood markers?**
- What habits do I need to **focus on now** so I don't slide back?
- How do **I make this work for me for the long haul?**

It's a **huge mental shift** to go from How do I survive this? to How do I build on this?

It's not just about losing weight anymore—it's about evolving into the version of myself who knows how to sustain it.

That means:

✔ **Leaving behind old habits.**

✔ **Rewriting the way I think about food, movement, and health.**

✔ **Deciding that my future is mine to shape.**

And yes—**this is way easier said than done.** But I truly believe that **awareness, attention, and intention are what create lasting change.**

Maybe that's why this week has felt so different—it's the first time I've thought about this journey as something that goes beyond just weight loss. **It's not just about numbers on the scale—it's about who I am becoming.**

(Also… this sounds like the **beginning of a new book.** 😄)

Biggest Takeaway of the Week?

I've started wanting things for my **health and my life** that I *never* thought were possible before.

💡 **New ideas about food.**

💡 **New approaches to movement and exercise.**

💡 **New routines for sleep, recovery, and overall well-being.**

Somewhere along the way, I had started to believe that **these things just weren't for me.**

That once I hit **53,** my ability to **change, grow, and redefine my health, my business, my relationships was limited.**

Turns out? **That was a lie.**

I can change. I am changing. And I have no idea where this journey will take me next.

But I can't wait to find out.

Week 15 Takeaways:

✔ **I've lost 25 pounds!** 🥳

✔ **Confidence isn't just about looks—it's about feeling at home in my body as well as my mind.**

✔ **My brain still thinks I need more food than I do. (Work in progress.)**

✔ **Alcohol? Meh. Sweets? Still tempting but manageable.**

✔ **The real work now is making this journey sustainable.**

Tirzepatide Times: Week 16 – The Unexpected Bonus & Finding My Balance

You know that moment when you realize you forgot to mention something huge? Like, life-changingly huge? Yeah, that's me right now.

So, rewind a few weeks—I casually left out a major "good" side effect of this whole Tirzepatide journey: I STOPPED SNORING.

This might not sound like a big deal, but if you've ever been the source of relentless nighttime noise pollution (guilty), you know how annoying, embarrassing, and relationship-wrecking snoring can be.

I've been snoring for over 10 years, to the point where my partner—who is a patient, loving, wonderful human—would sometimes have to wave the white flag and retreat to the guest room just to get some sleep. Not exactly ideal for a new relationship. And while she was kind about it, let's be real—it made me feel awful.

Then, a few weeks into my Tirzepatide adventure, she casually mentioned, "Hey, you haven't been snoring."

Excuse me, what?!

I couldn't believe it. Had I really gone from full-on freight train mode to silent sleeper? I asked her if she was sure, and she doubled down: "Not a peep."

Naturally, I've checked in a few times since (because, let's be honest, this is a game-changer), and she still says she hasn't heard me snore in weeks. Bonus side effect unlocked!

Week 16: The Routine Feels Solid

Beyond my newfound ability to sleep like a normal person, everything else feels pretty stable at this point. The unpredictable side effects have mostly settled, my energy is up, and I'm not feeling like I'm riding an emotional rollercoaster every week.

Life feels manageable. Health is on the upswing. And honestly? This medication is proving to be the miracle it was promised to be.

Of course, I know there are no guarantees for future use. I know my body is still adapting, and there's still so much to learn about these meds. But I have to admit—I'm fascinated by the process and by all the new research coming out.

The Next Phase: Finding Balance Again

Now that my body feels like it's in a good place, I'm shifting my focus toward:

✔ Getting back to being more active – Not just walking, but building real strength again.

✔ Enjoying food in moderation – Because food is meant to be enjoyed, not feared.

✔ Figuring out what confidence & health look like in this new phase of my life – Less about the number on the scale and more about how I feel.

I'll keep blogging and Instagramming my experiences because if I've learned anything from this journey, it's that talking about it helps—both for me and for anyone else considering this path.

For now, 16 weeks in, I can confidently say this experiment is paying off. I'm lighter (27 pounds in 16 weeks), healthier, happier—and apparently, a much quieter sleeper. 😉

6

THE INTEGRATION STRATEGY: COMBINING MEDICATIONS WITH LIFESTYLE CHANGES

Success with weight loss medications isn't about passive reliance on pills - it's about creating a powerful synergy between pharmaceutical support and lifestyle modifications. When I started Zepbound, I quickly realized that the medication wasn't a replacement for healthy habits, but rather a tool that made those habits easier to maintain and more effective. The journey through medical weight loss requires a thoughtful integration of both pharmaceutical support and lifestyle modifications - a delicate dance that, when mastered, can lead to transformative results. Through my own experience and countless conversations with others on similar paths, I've discovered that success lies not in viewing these medications as magic solutions, but as powerful tools that can amplify the effectiveness of healthy lifestyle choices.

Many people approach weight loss medications with the misconception that the medicine alone will do all the work. However, the most successful outcomes consistently come from those who embrace a comprehensive approach that includes:

- Strategic meal planning and portion control
- Regular physical activity tailored to individual capabilities
- Stress management techniques
- Consistent sleep patterns
- Strong support systems

The synergy between medication and lifestyle changes creates a powerful foundation for sustainable weight management. When the medication helps control appetite and cravings, it becomes easier to implement and maintain healthy eating habits. Similarly, when the body responds more efficiently to exercise due to improved metabolic function, maintaining an active lifestyle becomes more rewarding and sustainable.

Six months into my weight loss journey, I found myself at a crossroads during a family vacation in Maine. The medication had helped me lose weight, but now I faced the challenge of maintaining my new habits while away from my routine. One morning, I decided to turn this challenge into an opportunity. I woke up early, took my medication as scheduled, and instead of joining the family's traditional heavy breakfast, I packed a light, protein-rich meal and invited everyone for a beach walk. To my surprise, this sparked a transformation in our family dynamics. My sister-in-law, inspired by how I was balancing medication with lifestyle changes, started asking questions about my journey. By the end of the vacation, we had created a new family tradition of morning walks and mindful meals. This experience taught me that the real power of weight loss medications lies not in the pills themselves, but in how they can catalyze and support broader lifestyle changes. The medication gave me the initial boost I needed, but it was the integration of new habits and routines that made the changes sustainable.

Understanding this crucial relationship between medication and lifestyle modification opens the door to creating lasting change. Throughout this chapter, we'll explore practical strategies for maximizing the benefits of weight loss medications through thoughtful lifestyle integration. We'll examine how timing your medication, meals, and exercise can enhance results, and discuss ways to build sustainable habits that continue long after the medication journey ends.

The key to success lies in viewing weight loss medications not as a crutch, but as a scaffold - a temporary support structure that allows you to build stronger, healthier habits. As we delve deeper into these strategies, you'll discover how to create your own personalized approach that combines the benefits of medical intervention with sustainable lifestyle changes.

Timing Matters: Coordinating Medication, Meals, and Exercise for Maximum Effect

One of the most crucial aspects of successful weight loss medication use is understanding the intricate dance between timing your medication, meals, and physical activity. When I first started Zepbound, I quickly learned that random timing could lead to unnecessary side effects or reduced effectiveness. Through careful observation and adjustment, I discovered that strategic timing could make a significant difference in both results and comfort.

The timing of medication administration plays a vital role in maximizing its effectiveness while minimizing potential side effects. Here are the key timing considerations that can enhance your weight loss journey:

- Take medication at the same time each day to maintain consistent levels in your system
- Allow 30-60 minutes between medication and your first meal
- Plan exercise sessions when medication effects are strongest
- Space meals 4-6 hours apart to align with medication's appetite-suppressing effects
- Consider your daily schedule when choosing morning or evening dosing

Creating a consistent daily routine around these timing elements helps establish a rhythm that your body can adapt to. I found that keeping a simple timing log during my first month helped me identify patterns and adjust my schedule for optimal results.

The relationship between medication timing and meal planning deserves special attention. When I first started, I made the mistake of trying to maintain my old eating schedule. However, I soon realized that aligning my meals with the medication's peak effectiveness periods made a significant difference. A protein-rich breakfast about an hour after taking my medication helped stabilize my energy levels throughout the morning. Lunch and dinner then naturally fell into place around the medication's rhythm.

Exercise timing also plays a crucial role in maximizing the benefits of weight loss medications. Through trial and error, I discovered that moderate exercise during peak medication hours helped amplify the positive effects while reducing any potential gastrointestinal discomfort. Here's what I found works best:

- Light cardio or walking 1-2 hours after medication
- Strength training during mid-day when energy levels are stable

- Gentle evening activities like yoga or stretching
- Avoiding intense exercise immediately after taking medication
- Planning rest days when adjusting to new dosages

The key is to listen to your body and adjust these timing recommendations to fit your personal response to the medication. Everyone's body chemistry is unique, and what works perfectly for one person might need adjustment for another. I started keeping a simple journal noting how I felt at different times of day, which helped me fine-tune my schedule for optimal results.

Water intake timing also deserves careful consideration when taking weight loss medications. Staying well-hydrated helps minimize side effects and supports the medication's effectiveness. I developed a habit of drinking a full glass of water with my medication and then spacing additional water intake throughout the day, being careful not to drink too much right before or during meals.

Remember that timing optimization is an ongoing process. As your body adapts to the medication and your lifestyle changes, you may need to adjust your timing strategy. Pay attention to how your body responds and be willing to make modifications. The goal is to find a sustainable rhythm that works with your daily life while maximizing the benefits of your weight loss medication.

One particularly effective strategy I discovered was creating a timing map for each day. This visual guide helped me coordinate medication, meals, and exercise in a way that felt natural rather than forced. I started with the fixed point of my medication time and built the rest of my schedule around that anchor. This approach made it easier to maintain consistency while still allowing for the flexibility that real life demands.

Building Sustainable Habits: Using Medication Support to Establish Lasting Lifestyle Changes

The true power of weight loss medications lies in their ability to create a window of opportunity for establishing lasting healthy habits. During my journey with Zepbound, I discovered that the medication's appetite-suppressing effects provided the perfect environment to rewire my relationship with food and build sustainable lifestyle practices. This period of reduced hunger and cravings became my training ground for developing habits that would serve me well beyond my medication journey.

The key to building sustainable habits while on weight loss medication involves understanding the three crucial elements of habit formation:

- Trigger: The cue that initiates a behavior
- Action: The behavior itself
- Reward: The positive outcome that reinforces the behavior

Weight loss medications help by temporarily removing many of the physical and hormonal barriers that typically make habit formation challenging. For instance, when intense hunger signals no longer drive impulsive eating, you can thoughtfully establish new mealtime routines.

One afternoon in my kitchen, I had an enlightening moment while preparing lunch. Instead of my old habit of mindlessly grazing while cooking, I found myself naturally portioning out my meal and sitting down to eat without any internal struggle. The medication had created space for me to develop this new habit without fighting against overwhelming hunger signals. This experience showed me how medication support could serve as a scaffold for building lasting behavioral changes.

To maximize the habit-building potential of your medication journey, consider implementing these foundational practices:

- Create consistent meal timing routines

- Establish portion control systems
- Develop mindful eating practices
- Build regular physical activity patterns
- Design stress management techniques

The key is to use the medication's effects as a training period for these new habits. Think of it like learning to ride a bike with training wheels - the medication provides temporary support while you develop the balance and strength needed for long-term success.

I developed a simple habit-stacking approach that proved particularly effective. Each week, I would introduce one new small habit that built upon existing routines. For example, I started by placing a glass of water next to my coffee maker each evening. This simple action meant I automatically drank water first thing in the morning before my coffee. Once that became automatic, I added a short stretching routine while the coffee brewed.

The medication support makes this habit-building process significantly more manageable by:

- Reducing the physical and mental energy needed to establish new patterns
- Providing a period of reduced cravings to develop healthy food relationships
- Creating space for mindful decision-making around food and exercise
- Allowing for gradual, sustainable change rather than drastic measures

Tracking these developing habits becomes crucial for long-term success. I created a simple habit tracker in my phone that helped me monitor my progress and identify patterns. This data became invaluable as I worked with my healthcare provider to adjust my medication dosage and eventually plan for life after medication.

Remember that sustainable habits need to be realistic and adaptable to your lifestyle. While the medication provides support, focusing on developing habits that you can maintain even after completing your medication journey will help you create lasting change. This might mean starting with smaller, manageable changes rather than attempting dramatic lifestyle overhauls.

One particularly effective strategy involves creating environmental supports for your new habits. For instance, I reorganized my kitchen to make healthy food preparation easier and removed trigger foods from easily accessible locations. These physical changes helped reinforce my new habits even as the medication's effects fluctuated.

The goal is to use your time on medication to establish a foundation of healthy habits that will sustain your progress long-term. Think of this period as your opportunity to practice and cement these new behaviors while you have additional support from the medication. By focusing on habit formation during this time, you're investing in sustainable change rather than temporary solutions.

As you progress in your journey, regularly assess your habits and adjust as needed. What works in the beginning might need modification as your lifestyle or circumstances change. The key is to remain flexible while maintaining the core principles of healthy living you've established during your medication-supported period.

The Accountability Framework: Creating Support Systems and Progress Tracking Methods

Creating lasting change on your weight loss journey requires more than just willpower - it demands a robust system of accountability and support. Through my experience with Zepbound and working with numerous individuals on similar paths, I've discovered that those who build strong accountability frameworks are significantly more likely to achieve and maintain their goals.

Accountability in weight management operates on multiple levels, each playing a vital role in long-term success. The key elements of an effective accountability system include:

- Regular check-ins with healthcare providers
- Progress tracking tools and methods
- Support network engagement
- Clear milestone setting
- Consistent feedback mechanisms

One rainy Tuesday morning, I sat at my kitchen table reviewing my weight loss progress charts. Feeling discouraged by what seemed like a plateau, I realized I needed to revamp my accountability system. I reached out to my sister, who agreed to become my weekly check-in partner, and downloaded a comprehensive tracking app that would help me monitor not just weight, but also other important metrics like mood, energy levels, and sleep patterns.

The most effective progress tracking methods combine multiple data points to create a complete picture of your journey. Consider monitoring these key metrics:

- Body measurements beyond just weight
- Energy levels throughout the day
- Sleep quality and duration
- Medication timing and effects
- Exercise frequency and intensity
- Mood and stress levels
- Food choices and portion sizes

Building a strong support system is equally crucial for maintaining accountability. Your support network might include:

- Healthcare providers who understand your medication journey

- Family members or close friends who support your goals
- Online communities of others using similar medications
- Professional counselors or therapists
- Fitness instructors or personal trainers

The power of a well-structured accountability system became clear to me during a challenging family celebration. Having my sister as an accountability partner meant someone noticed when I started slipping into old habits. Her gentle reminder about my goals and the strategies we'd discussed helped me navigate the event while staying true to my weight management plan.

Tracking progress effectively requires choosing the right tools and methods for your lifestyle. Consider these practical tracking options:

- Digital health apps that sync with your devices
- Traditional paper journals or logs
- Photo documentation of meals and activities
- Weekly measurement records
- Progress photos at regular intervals

Establishing clear milestones helps break down your larger goals into manageable chunks. When setting milestones, consider both scale and non-scale victories:

- Weight loss targets at reasonable intervals
- Clothing size goals
- Fitness achievements
- Behavioral changes
- Medical marker improvements

The key to successful progress tracking is consistency and honesty. Create a daily routine that includes regular check-ins with your tracking system. This might mean spending five minutes each morning logging your weight and medication timing, or setting aside time each Sunday evening to plan the week ahead and review your progress.

One particularly effective strategy I've found is the "accountability triangle" - having three different types of support working together:

- Professional support (healthcare providers)
- Personal support (family/friends)
- Community support (support groups/online communities)

This three-pronged approach ensures you have support available in different contexts and for different needs. Your healthcare provider monitors medical progress, while friends and family offer emotional support, and community members share practical tips and experiences.

Remember that accountability systems need to evolve as your journey progresses. What works during the initial phases of medication may need adjustment as you develop new habits and face different challenges. Regular review and refinement of your accountability framework ensures it continues to serve your needs effectively.

Perhaps most importantly, your accountability system should celebrate progress while providing constructive feedback for areas needing improvement. This balanced approach helps maintain motivation without creating unnecessary pressure or anxiety about perfect adherence to your plan.

Creating weekly accountability rituals can help cement these practices into your routine. For instance, every Sunday evening, I review my week's data, plan for the upcoming week, and share updates with my accountability partner. This regular check-in provides structure and ensures I stay connected with my support system.

Your accountability framework should also include contingency plans for challenging situations. Having pre-planned strategies for handling setbacks or obstacles helps maintain progress even when facing unexpected challenges. This might include having backup exercise plans for bad weather or strategies for managing social events where food choices might be limited.

The journey of integrating weight loss medications with lifestyle changes is much like learning to dance - it requires practice, patience, and the right partnership between medical support and personal effort. Throughout this chapter, we've explored how medications can serve as powerful allies in establishing sustainable health habits, but only when combined with thoughtful lifestyle modifications.

The key lessons from this chapter highlight the essential elements of successful integration:

- Strategic timing of medication, meals, and exercise maximizes benefits while minimizing side effects
- Building sustainable habits during medication support creates lasting change
- Strong accountability frameworks and tracking systems enhance long-term success
- Support networks play a crucial role in maintaining motivation and consistency

My experience with Zepbound taught me that medication isn't just about controlling appetite - it's about creating a window of opportunity for transformative change. Those moments of reduced cravings become chances to establish new relationships with food. The increased energy becomes an invitation to develop consistent exercise routines. Each medication-supported day offers a chance to practice habits that will sustain long after the prescription ends.

Whether you're just beginning this journey or well along your path, remember that the real power lies not in the medication alone, but in how you use it to create meaningful, lasting change in your life. The strategies, timing techniques, and habit-building approaches we've explored provide a roadmap for making the most of this powerful tool while developing the skills and routines that will support your health for years to come.

7

MANAGING SIDE EFFECTS: WHAT TO EXPECT AND HOW TO COPE

Managing side effects from weight loss medications requires a delicate balance of patience, preparation, and proactive strategies. Like learning to drive a new car, understanding how your body responds to these medications takes time, but with the right knowledge and tools, you can navigate the adjustment period successfully. The reality is that every medication, no matter how beneficial, comes with potential side effects that need to be understood and managed effectively. Like many others on my weight management journey, I've learned that success isn't just about taking the medication - it's about developing strategies to handle the challenges that may arise along the way.

Three months into my Zepbound journey, I faced my biggest challenge during an important business presentation. Despite carefully timing my medication, I experienced unexpected nausea just before the meeting began. Drawing on the coping strategies I'd developed, I quickly sipped ginger tea and took slow, deep breaths. I had prepared for this possibility by eating a light, protein-rich breakfast and keeping anti-nausea drops in my briefcase.

The presentation went smoothly, and afterward, a colleague who was also on weight loss medication noticed my strategic approach. We began sharing our experiences and coping mechanisms, eventually creating an informal support group at work. This experience taught me that success with these medications isn't just about managing side effects - it's about developing a comprehensive toolkit of strategies that allow you to maintain your normal life while adapting to the medication's side effects. Through careful planning and the right coping techniques, what started as a challenging situation became an opportunity to help others navigate their own side effect management journey.

Understanding and preparing for potential side effects is crucial for anyone considering or currently taking weight loss medications. While these medications can be transformative for many people, being well-informed about what to expect and how to respond can make the difference between giving up in frustration and achieving lasting success. This chapter will equip you with practical strategies for managing common side effects, recognizing warning signs that require medical attention, and maintaining your quality of life while on these medications.

The key to successful side effect management lies in three essential approaches:

- Preparation and prevention
- Early recognition and response
- Consistent communication with healthcare providers

As we explore these topics in detail, you'll learn not just about potential side effects, but more importantly, how to develop your own personalized management strategy. Whether you're just starting your medication journey or looking to better manage existing side effects, this chapter will provide you with the tools and knowledge needed to navigate these challenges successfully. Remember that experiencing side effects doesn't mean the medication isn't right for you - it often means your body is adjusting to significant changes in how it processes food and manages appetite signals. Let's begin with understanding the most common side effects and how to prepare for them effectively.

Common Side Effects: Understanding and Preparing for Gastrointestinal Issues and Other Reactions

Gastrointestinal side effects are among the most common challenges faced by people taking weight loss medications, particularly GLP-1 agonists. During my first few weeks on Zepbound, I quickly learned that understanding and preparing for these effects wasn't just helpful - it was essential for success. While these side effects can be uncomfortable, they're often manageable with the right strategies and support.

The most frequently reported gastrointestinal side effects include:

- Nausea and occasional vomiting
- Changes in bowel movements (constipation or diarrhea)
- Bloating and gas

- Reduced appetite
- Stomach cramping

While these effects might sound daunting, remember that they're typically most pronounced during the initial weeks of treatment and often improve as your body adjusts to the medication. The key is having a solid management plan in place before you begin treatment.

One morning, about two weeks into my treatment, I experienced an unexpected wave of nausea during my daily commute. Thankfully, I had prepared for this possibility by keeping a 'side effect toolkit' in my car and office. This preparation made all the difference between a difficult day and a manageable one. Over time, I refined my approach based on what worked best for my body and schedule.

Here are proven strategies for managing gastrointestinal side effects:

- Eat smaller, more frequent meals throughout the day
- Stay well-hydrated with water and electrolyte beverages
- Avoid fatty or spicy foods, especially during the first few weeks
- Keep ginger tea or candies handy for nausea relief
- Time medications consistently with meals as directed by your healthcare provider

Beyond gastrointestinal effects, some people may experience other reactions that deserve attention. These can include:

- Headaches
- Fatigue
- Dizziness
- Injection site reactions (for injectable medications)
- Changes in taste preferences

The intensity and duration of side effects can vary significantly from person to person. What causes significant discomfort for one individual might be barely noticeable for another. This is why maintaining open communication with your healthcare provider is crucial - they can help adjust your treatment plan based on your specific experiences.

During my support group meetings, I've noticed that those who approach side effects with a proactive mindset tend to have more success with their treatment. Rather than viewing side effects as obstacles, they see them as signals that the medication is working and their body is adapting to a new way of processing food and managing hunger.

Keeping a side effect journal during your first few months of treatment can be invaluable. Track not only the effects you experience but also what strategies help manage them effectively. This information can help your healthcare provider optimize your treatment plan and provide insights for adjusting your daily routines.

Remember that while side effects are common, they shouldn't significantly impact your quality of life. If you find that side effects are becoming overwhelming, don't hesitate to discuss this with your healthcare provider. Sometimes, simple adjustments to dosing or timing can make a substantial difference in your experience.

Through my own journey and conversations with others, I've learned that successful side effect management often comes down to three key principles: preparation, patience, and persistence. By understanding what to expect and having strategies ready to implement, you can navigate this aspect of treatment with greater confidence and comfort.

The goal isn't to eliminate side effects entirely - that's often unrealistic. Instead, focus on developing effective management strategies that allow you to maintain your normal activities while your body adjusts to the medication. With time and proper support, most people find that side effects become more manageable, allowing them to focus on their weight management goals rather than the challenges of treatment.

Strategic Management: Practical Solutions for Minimizing Discomfort and Maintaining Quality of Life

Successfully managing side effects while maintaining your quality of life requires a strategic approach that goes beyond just treating symptoms as they arise. Through my experience with Zepbound and conversations with countless others on similar medications, I've discovered that the most successful patients are those who develop comprehensive management plans that fit seamlessly into their daily routines.

Here are key strategies for minimizing discomfort while maintaining your normal activities:

- Time your medications strategically around your schedule
- Keep a "rescue kit" of comfort items readily available
- Develop meal plans that work with your medication timing
- Create backup plans for important events and meetings
- Establish clear communication channels with your support network

One afternoon, while preparing for an important family wedding, I realized how far I'd come in managing my medication's side effects. Instead of worrying about potential nausea or fatigue during the celebration, I had a clear plan in place. I adjusted my medication timing slightly, packed my trusted ginger candies, and had already discussed menu options with the caterer. This preparation allowed me to fully enjoy the special day without anxiety about potential side effects.

Developing your personal comfort strategy should include:

- A daily schedule that aligns medication, meals, and activities
- Quick-relief solutions for common side effects
- Alternative plans for social situations and dining out
- Regular check-ins with your healthcare provider

- Exercise routines adapted to your energy levels

The key to maintaining quality of life while managing side effects lies in proactive planning rather than reactive responses. Consider creating a side effect management toolkit that includes:

- Anti-nausea remedies (ginger tea, candies, or prescribed medications)
- Portable snacks that work well with your medication
- Water bottle and electrolyte supplements
- Comfort items specific to your needs
- Emergency contact information

Learning to read your body's signals and respond appropriately takes time, but it's an essential skill for long-term success. Pay attention to patterns in how your body reacts to different foods, activities, and stress levels. This awareness will help you adjust your management strategies effectively.

For workplace success, consider these practical solutions:

- Schedule important meetings during your peak hours
- Keep emergency supplies discretely stored at your desk
- Inform key colleagues about your medication journey if comfortable
- Plan ahead for business travel or long meetings
- Have backup plans for unexpected situations

Social situations require their own set of strategies. I've found success with:

- Reviewing restaurant menus in advance
- Eating a small, safe meal before social events
- Having prepared responses for food-related questions

- Identifying safe food options at regular venues
- Planning medication timing around social events

Remember that maintaining quality of life isn't just about managing physical symptoms - it's also about preserving your emotional and social well-being. Don't let side effect management isolate you from activities and relationships you enjoy. Instead, use these strategies to adapt and thrive.

One particularly effective approach I've developed is the "15-minute rule." When experiencing discomfort, wait 15 minutes before taking action. Often, side effects are temporary and will pass on their own. This simple strategy has helped me avoid overreacting to minor discomfort while still being prepared for more persistent issues.

For long-term success, establish regular check-ins with yourself to assess:

- Overall effectiveness of your management strategies
- Impact on daily activities and relationships
- Need for adjustments to your approach
- Progress toward your health goals
- Quality of life satisfaction

Don't hesitate to adjust your strategies as needed. What works during the initial adjustment period might need modification as your body adapts to the medication. Stay flexible and open to refining your approach based on experience.

Most importantly, remember that managing side effects shouldn't become the central focus of your life. The goal is to develop efficient, effective strategies that run in the background, allowing you to focus on your weight management journey and overall well-being. With proper planning and the right tools in place, you can maintain your quality of life while working toward your health goals.

Red Flags and Emergency Signals: When to Contact Your Healthcare Provider

While most side effects of weight loss medications are manageable, there are certain warning signs that require immediate medical attention. Understanding these red flags can help you distinguish between normal adjustment symptoms and potentially serious complications. My own experience with Zepbound taught me the vital importance of knowing when to reach out to healthcare providers, and how quick action can prevent minor issues from becoming major concerns.

Here are the urgent warning signs that require immediate medical attention:

- Severe or persistent abdominal pain that doesn't improve
- Unusual heart palpitations or racing heartbeat
- Severe headache accompanied by vision changes
- Signs of allergic reaction (rash, swelling, difficulty breathing)
- Persistent vomiting or severe dehydration
- Unusual mood changes or thoughts of self-harm
- Severe injection site reactions (for injectable medications)

One evening during my third month of treatment, I experienced unusual heart palpitations that felt different from typical medication side effects. Instead of dismissing it or waiting to see if it would pass, I contacted my healthcare provider's after-hours line. While it turned out to be a temporary reaction to combining my medication with too much caffeine, the experience reinforced the importance of erring on the side of caution when unusual symptoms arise.

The development of certain symptoms may indicate a need to adjust or pause your medication. Contact your healthcare provider promptly if you experience:

- Persistent nausea that significantly impacts daily activities

- Unexplained changes in blood sugar levels (especially for diabetic patients)
- New or worsening depression or anxiety
- Severe constipation lasting more than three days
- Unusual swelling in arms or legs
- Persistent fatigue that interferes with daily activities

Severe dehydration is a side effect that needs to be urgently addressed. Signs of severe dehydration that warrant immediate attention include:

- Dark-colored urine or decreased urination
- Extreme thirst
- Dizziness or lightheadedness when standing
- Dry mouth and lips
- Decreased skin elasticity
- Unusual fatigue or confusion

I maintain a simple system for evaluating symptoms using what I call the '3-3-3 Rule': If a side effect lasts more than 3 hours (for acute symptoms), occurs more than 3 times in a row, or persists for more than 3 days (for ongoing issues), it's time to contact your healthcare provider.

Keep detailed records of any concerning symptoms, including:

- When the symptom started
- How long it lasts
- What makes it better or worse
- Any recent changes in medication or routine
- Other medications or supplements you're taking

This information helps your healthcare provider make informed decisions about your treatment plan. Remember, it's better to make an unnecessary call than to ignore a potentially serious situation.

Create an emergency contact list that includes:

- Your primary healthcare provider's office number
- After-hours or emergency contact information
- Local urgent care facilities
- Pharmacy contact information
- A trusted family member or friend

Store this information in your phone and keep a written copy in your wallet or purse. When in doubt about the severity of a symptom, consider this simple question: 'Is this different from my usual medication side effects?' If the answer is yes, it's worth reaching out to your healthcare provider.

Don't hesitate to advocate for yourself if you feel something isn't right. During my weight loss journey, I learned that being proactive about health concerns isn't just about safety - it's about optimizing your treatment success. Your healthcare provider would rather hear from you early about a potential issue than deal with complications that could have been prevented.

Remember that certain medications may interact with weight loss drugs, potentially causing adverse effects. Always inform your healthcare provider about:

- New prescriptions from other doctors
- Over-the-counter medications
- Herbal supplements or vitamins
- Changes in existing medication dosages

By staying vigilant about potential warning signs while maintaining open communication with your healthcare team, you can ensure a safer and more successful weight management journey. Trust your instincts - if something feels significantly wrong, it's always better to seek professional guidance than to wait and wonder.

As we conclude our exploration of side effect management, it's clear that success with weight loss medications isn't just about enduring challenges - it's about developing smart strategies to thrive while reaching your health goals.

Throughout this chapter, we've examined the common side effects, practical management approaches, and crucial warning signs that require medical attention. The strategies and insights shared here form a foundation for a more comfortable and successful medication journey.

Key takeaway points from this chapter include:

- Most side effects are manageable with proper preparation and strategy
- Early intervention and proactive planning make a significant difference
- Having a support system and emergency plan in place is crucial
- Regular communication with healthcare providers ensures optimal treatment
- Quality of life can be maintained while managing side effects

As you move forward with your weight management journey, remember that experiencing side effects doesn't mean failure - it's often a sign that your body is adjusting to positive changes. The key is developing personalized strategies that work for your lifestyle while staying vigilant about potential warning signs.

Your next steps should focus on:

- Creating your personal side effect management toolkit
- Establishing clear communication channels with your healthcare team
- Developing contingency plans for various situations

- Building a support network that understands your journey
- Keeping detailed records of your experiences and successful strategies

My own journey with Zepbound taught me that managing side effects is both an art and a science. It requires patience, preparation, and persistence, but the results are worth the effort. As you continue your weight management journey, use the strategies and insights from this chapter to create your own success story.

Remember, each person's experience with weight loss medications is unique. What works perfectly for one person might need adjustment for another. Stay flexible in your approach, maintain open communication with your healthcare providers, and trust your instincts about your body's signals. With the right preparation and mindset, side effects can become manageable challenges rather than insurmountable obstacles.

As we move into the next chapter, we'll explore how to maintain your success over the long term, building on the foundation of effective side effect management to create sustainable results. The skills you've learned here will serve as valuable tools throughout your weight management journey, helping you navigate challenges while staying focused on your health goals.

BONUS ARTICLE ON THE MICRO-DOSING GLP-1 TREND

What is GLP1 Micro-Dosing and Why Should We Care?

I am constantly researching and reading about the latest GLP1 information, and I came across an article in [The Hollywood Reporter] that made me pause. I read the article several times in amazement, and then I did some research. What I have written here is just a tiny scratch of the surface, but I found it fascinating, and I wonder if it is potentially an even more amazing discovery than anyone thought, or just another flash in the pan. Here is a taste of what I discovered, but take some time if you are interested and do your own research.

In the buzzing wellness circles of Los Angeles, there's always a new trend catching fire—and right now, that trend is GLP-1 micro-dosing. Originally intended for managing type 2 diabetes and chronic obesity, GLP-1 medications like Semaglutide and Tirzepatide have become incredibly popular, gaining traction among those looking for subtler, manageable results without the typical side effects of higher doses. But what exactly is micro-dosing GLP-1, and why has it become the latest must-try in LA's health-conscious communities?

What is GLP-1 Micro-dosing?

GLP-1, or glucagon-like peptide-1, medications traditionally help regulate blood sugar, suppress appetite, and facilitate weight loss when used at therapeutic doses. However, these higher dosages often come with noticeable side effects like nausea, fatigue, and gastrointestinal discomfort. Micro-dosing involves taking significantly smaller, carefully measured amounts, aiming to reap benefits such as mild appetite suppression, improved metabolic markers, and gradual weight management, without the harsh side effects.

Why LA is Embracing Micro-dosing

Los Angeles is a city famously obsessed with wellness, fitness, and aesthetics, often setting trends that ripple through the rest of the world. The allure of GLP-1 micro-dosing aligns perfectly with LA's ethos: a desire for subtle enhancement rather than dramatic changes that come with unwanted physical consequences.

"Micro-dosing appeals to people who are generally healthy but feel they need just a bit of help controlling cravings or shedding those stubborn last few pounds," explains Dr. Clara Nguyen, an endocrinologist based in Beverly Hills. "Many of my patients are attracted to the idea of gradual, gentle change without experiencing debilitating side effects."

How Does GLP-1 Micro-dosing Work?

Micro-dosing GLP-1 medication typically involves taking around one-quarter to one-third of a standard prescribed dose. The lower dosage gently influences hunger signals, metabolic regulation, and insulin sensitivity. The effect is more subtle—users might notice feeling full more quickly or experiencing reduced cravings, particularly for sugars and carbohydrates.

Sophia, a 32-year-old marketing executive in Venice, shared her experience: "I've never struggled significantly with weight, but after hitting 30, my metabolism shifted. A friend introduced me to micro-dosing semaglutide, and I noticed I didn't obsess over food as much. I felt satisfied with smaller portions, and within a few months, I effortlessly dropped about eight pounds."

Benefits and Potential Drawbacks

Benefits:

- Reduced side effects compared to standard dosages.
- Subtle appetite control aids mindful eating habits.
- Gradual weight loss and improved metabolic health.

Drawbacks:

- Lack of extensive long-term research on micro-dosing efficacy.
- Potential misuse without professional guidance.
- Still relatively expensive without insurance coverage.

Experts warn that despite its lower doses, micro-dosing is not without risks. "People might underestimate the potency of these medications," cautions Dr. Nguyen. "Even small doses should be overseen by healthcare providers to ensure proper monitoring and safety."

The Importance of Professional Guidance

The rising popularity of GLP-1 micro-dosing in LA has created a booming demand, sometimes bypassing traditional medical channels. However, medical professionals stress the importance of working closely with a healthcare provider.

"These medications are powerful tools," says Dr. Carlos Mendoza, an LA-based internist. "Micro-dosing isn't just about taking less medication; it's about precision and understanding your body's unique response. Medical oversight helps avoid pitfalls and ensures you achieve the health outcomes you're looking for safely."

A Trend With Staying Power?

While GLP-1 micro-dosing has gained rapid popularity in LA, especially within wellness and entertainment circles, only time and research will confirm its long-term benefits and sustainability. Still, anecdotal experiences like Sophia's are fueling interest, particularly among individuals aiming for moderation rather than transformation.

In a city where health trends come and go, GLP-1 micro-dosing seems uniquely positioned to stay. It offers a compelling blend of moderation, subtlety, and noticeable benefits without dramatic downsides.

Broader Therapeutic Potential of GLP-1 RAs

Emerging research suggests that GLP-1 receptor agonists (GLP-1 RAs), like semaglutide and liraglutide, offer therapeutic benefits beyond diabetes and obesity, potentially addressing addiction and neurodegenerative diseases like Alzheimer's and Parkinson's.

Addiction Treatment Potential

Preclinical studies have found that GLP-1 RAs can influence the brain's reward pathways involved in addiction by modulating dopamine signaling. These drugs could reduce the reinforcing effects of substances like alcohol and drugs, potentially easing withdrawal symptoms and reducing relapse risks. However, comprehensive clinical trials are essential to confirm these benefits conclusively.

Neurodegenerative Diseases

- Alzheimer's Disease: Animal studies have shown that GLP-1 RAs exhibit neuroprotective effects, improving cognitive functions and reducing Alzheimer's hallmark pathologies like amyloid plaques and neurofibrillary tangles. Mechanisms may involve improved insulin signaling in the brain, reduced inflammation, and enhanced neuronal survival. Notably, recent findings from the Alzheimer's Association International Conference (AAIC) 2024 indicated that liraglutide might slow cognitive decline by up to 18% over one year in mild Alzheimer's patients.

- Parkinson's Disease: GLP-1 RAs have demonstrated neuroprotective benefits in animal models of Parkinson's Disease by restoring dopamine levels, preventing neuron loss, and alleviating motor deficits. These effects may result from reduced inflammation, oxidative stress, and mitochondrial dysfunction. However, a notable 2025 study in The Lancet found exenatide did not significantly slow disease progression in Parkinson's patients over 96 weeks.

Anti-Inflammatory Properties

Additionally, GLP-1 RAs exhibit anti-inflammatory properties that might further contribute to their potential in neurodegenerative diseases by slowing neuroinflammation. Thus, they could potentially improve neuronal health and slow disease progression.

Conclusion

Expanding research underscores GLP-1 receptor agonists' potential beyond traditional uses. While early studies and community reports are encouraging, comprehensive clinical trials remain critical for validating micro-dosing as a safe, effective practice. For those navigating the wellness landscape, staying informed and prioritizing professional guidance will be key to leveraging this promising yet nuanced approach to health.

Resources

- [American Diabetes Association] (https://www.diabetes.org/)
- [Endocrine Society Guidelines on GLP-1 Medications] (https://www.endocrine.org/clinical-practice-guidelines)
- [National Institute of Diabetes and Digestive and Kidney Diseases (NIDDK)] (https://www.niddk.nih.gov/)
- [CDC Guidelines on Healthy Weight] (https://www.cdc.gov/healthyweight/index.html)

- [Los Angeles County Department of Public Health] (http://publichealth.lacounty.gov/)
- [PubMed Central] (https://pmc.ncbi.nlm.nih.gov/) for emerging research articles

8

THE LONG GAME: SUSTAINABLE SUCCESS AND LIFE AFTER MEDICATION

The true measure of success in weight management isn't just about reaching a goal weight - it's about maintaining those results through life's inevitable changes and challenges. As someone who has navigated both the peaks and valleys of this journey, I've learned that sustainable success requires a thoughtful strategy that extends far beyond the medication phase. The path to sustainable weight management extends far beyond simply reaching a target number on the scale. Like any significant life change, the journey requires careful planning, steadfast dedication, and the development of lasting habits that will serve as anchors through life's inevitable ups and downs.

Two years after starting my weight loss medication journey, I faced an unexpected challenge when my insurance coverage changed. Instead of panicking, I used this as an opportunity to test the strength of the habits and systems I'd built. I had spent months developing a morning routine that included protein-rich breakfasts, regular exercise, and stress management techniques. I'd also created a support network through my local wellness center and family members who understood my journey. During the three-month period while I worked to restore my medication coverage, I found that these established habits served as a sturdy bridge, helping me maintain most of my progress.

While I did experience some changes in appetite, the foundational lifestyle changes I'd implemented proved remarkably resilient. This experience taught me the vital importance of building sustainable habits alongside medication use, and how these habits become crucial anchors during life's inevitable transitions. When I eventually resumed my medication, I had a new appreciation for the complementary role it played in my overall wellness strategy, rather than seeing it as the sole solution.

This chapter explores the critical factors that determine long-term success in weight management, whether continuing with medication or transitioning to a medication-free approach. We'll examine proven strategies for maintaining results through various life stages and challenges, while addressing common concerns about life after active treatment. Most importantly, we'll focus on building the mental and emotional resilience necessary for sustainable weight management.

As we delve into the key components of successful long-term weight management, we'll explore how to weave them into a personalized strategy that works with your lifestyle, preferences, and goals. Whether you're currently on medication or planning for future transitions, this chapter will provide the tools and insights needed to build a sustainable approach to weight management that can last a lifetime.

The journey toward lasting weight management success is deeply personal, yet certain universal principles apply to everyone seeking to maintain their progress. By understanding these principles and learning to apply them effectively, you can develop a framework for success that endures well beyond your active medication phase.

Transition Planning: Strategies for Maintaining Success With or Without Continued Medication

One of the most crucial aspects of any weight management journey is developing a solid transition strategy, whether you plan to continue medication long-term or eventually discontinue it. The key lies in building a foundation of sustainable habits while the medication provides support, creating a safety net for whatever path you choose.

During my own journey with Zepbound, I learned that successful transition planning requires a methodical approach that begins long before any medication changes occur. The process starts with understanding your current patterns and gradually building systems that can function independently of medication support.

Essential elements of a successful transition plan include:

- Regular monitoring of eating patterns and hunger signals
- Established exercise routines that feel sustainable
- Strong stress management techniques

- A support network of healthcare providers and loved ones
- Clear triggers and action plans for potential setbacks

The transition process works best when approached in phases rather than as an abrupt change. Start by documenting your current routines, including meal timing, portion sizes, and exercise habits. This baseline information becomes invaluable as you begin making adjustments to your medication schedule or dosage.

I discovered the power of this approach when I needed to adjust my medication timing due to a schedule change at work. By having detailed records of my eating patterns and hunger cues, I could anticipate challenging periods and prepare accordingly. This experience taught me that successful transitions depend more on preparation and awareness than on willpower alone.

For those planning to continue medication long-term, transition planning focuses on optimizing the medication's benefits while building robust lifestyle habits. Key strategies include:

- Regular check-ins with healthcare providers to assess medication effectiveness
- Developing consistent meal planning and preparation routines
- Building a sustainable exercise program that adapts to life changes
- Creating backup plans for medication access issues

If you're considering discontinuing medication, the transition plan becomes even more critical. Start by working with your healthcare provider to develop a gradual tapering schedule that allows your body to adjust. During this period, pay extra attention to hunger signals and energy levels, adjusting your habits as needed.

Regardless of your chosen path, successful transition planning requires honest self-assessment and proactive problem-solving. Consider keeping a journal to track your progress and identify areas that need additional support. This documentation can help you and your healthcare team make informed decisions about your ongoing treatment plan.

One valuable strategy I've found is creating what I call 'success anchors' - specific habits or routines that remain constant regardless of medication status. These might include:

- A morning routine that includes movement and mindful eating
- Weekly meal prep sessions
- Regular check-ins with a support person or group
- Stress-management practices like meditation or journaling

Remember that transition planning isn't about preparing for an endpoint - it's about building a sustainable approach to health that can evolve with your needs. Think of it as creating a personal operating system for health that can run with or without medication support. Whether medication remains part of your long-term strategy or serves as a temporary tool, the habits and systems you develop during this phase will serve as the foundation for lasting success.

Perhaps most importantly, approach your transition with patience and self-compassion. Weight management is a journey, not a destination, and the most successful transitions are those that prioritize steady progress over quick results. By taking time to build strong foundations while medication provides support, you create the conditions for lasting success, regardless of your long-term treatment decisions.

Building Resilience: Preparing for Life Changes and Challenges While Maintaining Weight Loss

Life has a way of throwing unexpected challenges at us, especially during a weight management journey. Building resilience isn't just about handling these challenges - it's about developing the mental and emotional strength to maintain progress despite them. Through my experience with Zepbound and working with others on similar journeys,

I've learned that preparation and adaptability are key to long-term success.

Resilience in weight management encompasses several crucial elements:

- Emotional preparedness for setbacks and fluctuations
- Flexible strategies that adapt to changing circumstances
- Strong support systems that provide stability during challenges
- Clear action plans for common obstacles
- Self-compassion and realistic expectations

During my second year of weight management, a family emergency required me to become a temporary caregiver for my mother. The stress, disrupted routines, and emotional eating triggers threatened to derail my progress. However, the resilience strategies I had developed helped me maintain stability during this challenging period.

The experience taught me that resilience isn't about perfect adherence to a plan - it's about having the tools and mindset to navigate life's challenges while maintaining overall progress. This realization led me to develop what I call the 'Resilience Toolkit' - a personalized set of strategies for managing common challenges:

- Stress Management Techniques: Deep breathing exercises, short meditation sessions, or brief walks
- Meal Preparation Backups: Quick, healthy meal options for busy periods
- Exercise Alternatives: Modified workouts for different situations and energy levels
- Support Network Contacts: Key people to reach out to during challenging times

Building resilience requires anticipating potential challenges and preparing for them before they arise. Common life changes that can impact weight management include:

- Career transitions or job stress
- Family responsibilities and caregiving
- Financial changes affecting medication access
- Health challenges or injuries
- Major life events (moving, relationships, etc.)

For each potential challenge, develop specific strategies and backup plans. For instance, if you know work stress triggers emotional eating, create a list of alternative stress-relief activities. If travel disrupts your routine, prepare a travel-friendly exercise plan and identify healthy food options in advance.

One particularly effective approach is the 'Challenge-Strategy-Support' framework:

- Challenge: Identify potential obstacles
- Strategy: Develop specific action plans
- Support: Determine what resources and help you'll need

The key to building lasting resilience lies in viewing challenges as opportunities for growth rather than threats to progress. When I faced a three-week business trip that disrupted my usual routine, I used it as a chance to develop new strategies for maintaining healthy habits while traveling. Instead of seeing the trip as a setback, I treated it as a learning experience to strengthen my resilience toolkit.

Practical steps for building resilience include:

- Regular self-assessment of potential challenges
- Proactive planning for common obstacles
- Building a diverse support network
- Practicing flexible thinking and adaptability
- Developing multiple strategies for common situations

Remember that resilience grows stronger with each challenge you navigate successfully. Start by identifying your most likely challenges and developing specific strategies for each. Practice these strategies during stable periods so they become automatic responses when needed.

Maintaining progress during life changes also requires adjusting expectations while keeping sight of long-term goals. When I needed to modify my exercise routine due to a minor injury, I focused on what I could do rather than what I couldn't. This mindset helped maintain momentum while allowing necessary adjustments.

The most resilient weight management plans include:

- Multiple backup strategies for key habits
- Regular check-ins with healthcare providers
- Clear communication with support network members
- Flexible goals that adapt to changing circumstances
- Regular review and updating of strategies

By building these resilience factors into your weight management plan, you create a robust framework that can withstand life's inevitable challenges while maintaining progress toward your goals. Remember, resilience isn't about avoiding challenges - it's about having the tools and mindset to navigate them successfully while staying committed to your health journey.

Creating Your Forever Plan: Developing Sustainable Habits and Support Systems

Creating a sustainable weight management plan isn't about following a rigid set of rules - it's about developing a flexible framework that can evolve with your life while supporting your health goals. Through my experience with Zepbound and countless conversations with others on similar journeys, I've learned that lasting success comes from building what I call a 'Forever Plan' - a personalized approach that feels natural rather than forced.

The foundation of any Forever Plan rests on three key pillars:

- Sustainable daily habits that feel effortless
- Strong support systems that provide accountability and encouragement
- Flexible routines that can adapt to life's changes

One spring morning, I realized my Forever Plan was truly working when I automatically reached for my running shoes instead of hitting the snooze button. It wasn't willpower or obligation driving me - it had simply become part of who I am. This transformation didn't happen overnight, but through careful cultivation of habits that aligned with my lifestyle and preferences.

Creating your Forever Plan starts with honest self-assessment. Consider these essential elements:

- Your natural daily rhythms and energy patterns
- Food preferences and cooking abilities
- Available time for exercise and meal preparation
- Support resources in your community
- Personal stress management techniques that work for you

The key to developing sustainable habits lies in starting small and building gradually. Rather than overhauling your entire lifestyle at once, focus on implementing one change at a time until it becomes automatic. For instance, begin with establishing a consistent breakfast routine before tackling exercise habits.

Core components of a successful Forever Plan include:

- Regular movement that you genuinely enjoy
- Balanced eating patterns that satisfy both nutrition and pleasure

- Stress management techniques that fit your personality
- Social connections that support your health goals
- Regular self-monitoring practices

Building your support system requires thoughtful consideration and active cultivation. Identify people who can serve different roles in your journey:

- Healthcare providers for medical guidance
- Friends or family for emotional support
- Exercise partners for accountability
- Meal planning buddies for shared motivation
- Professional counselors or coaches when needed

My own Forever Plan took shape through careful experimentation and adjustment. I discovered that morning workouts suited my schedule better than evening sessions, and that preparing meals in advance prevented impulsive food choices. These weren't just temporary fixes - they became integral parts of my daily life.

Creating sustainable habits requires understanding the difference between discipline and automation. While discipline helps establish new behaviors, automation maintains them long-term. Focus on building habits that:

- Feel natural and enjoyable
- Fit seamlessly into your daily routine
- Provide immediate positive feedback
- Can be modified when circumstances change
- Support your overall well-being

Remember that your Forever Plan should be flexible enough to accommodate life's changes while maintaining core healthy habits. Think of it as a living document that evolves with you rather than a rigid set of rules.

Practical steps for developing your Forever Plan:

- Start with a weekly schedule audit to identify natural habit insertion points
- Choose one habit to focus on at a time
- Build in regular check-ins to assess progress
- Create backup plans for common obstacles
- Establish clear success metrics beyond the scale

The most successful Forever Plans include both structured elements and flexibility. For example, having set meal prep days while allowing for spontaneous social dining, or maintaining a regular exercise schedule while being open to trying new activities.

Your support system should grow and evolve alongside your habits. Consider:

- Joining local fitness or wellness groups
- Connecting with online communities
- Building relationships with healthcare providers
- Creating accountability partnerships
- Engaging family members in healthy activities

The goal isn't perfection but progress - creating a sustainable approach that supports long-term health while allowing for life's natural variations. Your Forever Plan should feel like a natural extension of who you are, not a constant battle against your inclinations.

Focus on progress over perfection, and be patient with yourself as you develop your Forever Plan. The most successful long-term weight management strategies are those that become so integrated into your lifestyle that they no longer feel like effort - they're simply part of who you are.

As we conclude this exploration of sustainable weight management and life after medication, it's clear that the journey doesn't end with reaching a goal weight or completing a medication cycle. The path forward requires thoughtful planning, resilience, and the development of lasting habits that can weather life's inevitable changes.

Through the stories and strategies shared in this chapter, we've seen how successful long-term weight management depends on several key factors:

- Building robust support systems that extend beyond healthcare providers
- Developing sustainable habits that feel natural rather than forced
- Creating flexible routines that can adapt to life's changes
- Establishing clear transition plans for medication adjustments
- Maintaining realistic expectations while staying committed to progress

The journey of weight management is deeply personal, yet certain universal truths emerge. Success isn't measured solely by numbers on a scale but by the quality of life improvements and sustainable habits we develop along the way. Whether continuing with medication or transitioning to a medication-free approach, the foundations built during this phase become crucial anchors for lasting success.

Take action today by:

- Documenting your current routines and identifying areas for improvement
- Creating a personal 'Resilience Toolkit' for managing common challenges
- Building connections with support resources in your community
- Developing backup plans for potential medication access issues
- Starting small with sustainable habit changes

Your Forever Plan should feel like a natural extension of who you are, not a constant battle against your inclinations. By focusing on building sustainable habits while medication provides support, you create the conditions for lasting success that can endure through life's inevitable changes and challenges.

As we conclude this chapter, consider how you'll apply these principles to your own journey. Start with small, manageable changes that align with your lifestyle and preferences. Remember that each step forward, no matter how small, contributes to your long-term success. The goal isn't to create a perfect plan but to develop a sustainable approach that can evolve with you while supporting your health and wellness goals.

Your weight management journey is uniquely yours, but you're not alone in this process. The strategies, tools, and insights shared in this chapter can serve as guideposts as you create your own path forward. Whether you're continuing with medication or planning for a future transition, focus on building the foundations that will support your long-term success.

Remember, this isn't the end of your story - it's the beginning of a new chapter in your ongoing journey toward sustainable wellness.

9 BIG PHARMA, BIG MONEY: THE ECONOMICS AND ETHICS OF WEIGHT LOSS DRUGS

Behind every breakthrough weight loss medication lies a complex web of financial decisions, market forces, and ethical considerations that shape not just the drug's development, but also who gets access to it. The intersection of profit and public health in the weight loss medication industry represents one of healthcare's most challenging ethical battlegrounds, where the promise of effective treatment often collides with the harsh realities of cost and accessibility.

The reality is that developing and bringing a new weight loss medication to market typically costs pharmaceutical companies hundreds of millions of dollars and takes over a decade of research, clinical trials, and regulatory reviews. This investment drives pricing decisions that can put these medications out of reach for many who could benefit from them.

During a routine pharmacy visit to refill my Zepbound prescription, I encountered Maria, a retired teacher who was carefully counting out cash from an envelope. She had been prescribed the same medication as me, but wasn't covered by insurance. As we chatted, she shared her struggle to afford the monthly cost, despite the medication's life-changing potential. This chance meeting inspired me to investigate patient assistance programs and alternative coverage options.

Over the next few weeks, I helped Maria navigate the complex world of pharmaceutical assistance programs, insurance appeals, and manufacturer discounts. Through this process, we uncovered a labyrinth of pricing tiers, coverage policies, and assistance programs that many patients never discover. Maria eventually secured coverage through a combination of manufacturer assistance and an insurance appeal, but our journey revealed the stark reality of how economic factors can create barriers to potentially life-changing medications. This experience highlighted the critical importance of understanding not just the medical aspects of weight loss drugs, but also the complex economic systems that determine who can access them.

The commercialization of weight loss solutions raises important questions about healthcare equity and corporate responsibility. While pharmaceutical companies must balance research investments and shareholder interests, the current pricing models have created a two-tiered system where access often depends more on economic status than medical need. Consider these key factors shaping the industry:

- Research and development costs drive high initial pricing
- Patent protection periods influence market competition
- Insurance coverage policies vary widely between providers
- Patient assistance programs have complex eligibility requirements
- Marketing expenditures impact final consumer costs

As we examine these market dynamics, we must consider both the tremendous potential these medications offer and the ethical implications of their current distribution model. The pharmaceutical industry's role in addressing obesity - now recognized as a chronic disease - comes with both opportunities and responsibilities. This chapter will explore how various stakeholders, from drug manufacturers to insurance companies to healthcare providers, influence who can access these potentially life-changing treatments.

Understanding these economic forces isn't just academic - it directly impacts treatment decisions and access to care. For patients considering weight loss medications, knowledge of the financial landscape can be as crucial as understanding the medical aspects. We'll explore strategies for navigating insurance coverage, finding assistance programs, and making informed decisions about treatment options within financial constraints.

The story of weight loss medications is ultimately about more than just profits and losses - it's about how society values and provides access to innovative medical treatments. As these medications become increasingly effective and in-demand, the pressure to create more equitable access systems continues to grow. Through examining this complex landscape, we can better understand both the challenges and potential solutions for making these treatments more accessible to all who need them.

The Cost of Innovation: Understanding Drug Development and Pricing

The journey of bringing a new weight loss medication from initial concept to pharmacy shelves is both lengthy and expensive. As I discovered while documenting my own experience with Zepbound, the price tag we see at the pharmacy counter reflects years of research, countless clinical trials, and rigorous safety testing. A typical weight loss medication takes 10-12 years to develop and can cost pharmaceutical companies between $800 million to over $2 billion before it ever reaches patients.

To understand why these medications come with such high price tags, let's break down the key stages of drug development:

- Initial Research and Discovery: Scientists must identify and test thousands of potential compounds
- Preclinical Testing: Laboratory and animal studies to assess safety and potential effectiveness
- Clinical Trials: Multiple phases of human testing involving thousands of participants
- FDA Review and Approval: Extensive documentation and safety verification process
- Post-Market Safety Monitoring: Ongoing studies and safety surveillance

One afternoon, while reviewing my medication costs with my insurance provider, I connected with Sarah, a clinical research coordinator who had worked on early trials for GLP-1 medications. She shared how for every successful drug that makes it to market, countless others fail during development - often after significant investment. These failed attempts are essentially built into the cost of successful medications, as pharmaceutical companies must recoup their total research investments to continue developing new treatments.

The pricing structure of weight loss medications reflects this complex development process. When a new drug first enters the market, pharmaceutical companies typically have exclusive rights to sell it for a limited time through patent protection. This period allows them to recoup their research investments before generic versions can be developed. However, this system creates a challenging balance between innovation and accessibility.

Key factors that influence the final cost of weight loss medications include:

- Research and development expenses
- Clinical trial costs
- Manufacturing and quality control
- Marketing and distribution
- Regulatory compliance requirements

Understanding these cost factors helps explain why newer medications like Wegovy or Zepbound often come with higher price tags than older weight loss drugs. The sophisticated technology behind these newer treatments - particularly their ability to target specific hormonal pathways - represents significant scientific advancement, but also increased development costs.

My own experience navigating insurance coverage for Zepbound revealed the complex relationship between drug pricing and access. While the list price was initially shocking, I learned about various programs that can help make these medications more affordable:

- Manufacturer savings cards and copay assistance programs
- Patient assistance programs for those without insurance
- Insurance formulary tiers and prior authorization processes
- Healthcare flexible spending accounts (FSAs) and health savings accounts (HSAs)

The investment in developing these medications continues to drive innovation in the field. Each new generation of weight loss drugs builds upon previous research, potentially offering improved effectiveness or reduced side effects. However, this ongoing innovation cycle also means continued high development costs that influence pricing.

For patients considering weight loss medications, understanding these economic factors can help inform decisions about treatment options. While the cost of newer medications may seem daunting, it's important to weigh them against potential health benefits and long-term medical cost savings. Working closely with healthcare providers and insurance companies to understand coverage options and assistance programs can help make these innovative treatments more accessible.

As we look to the future of weight loss medication development, the challenge remains: how do we balance the need for continued pharmaceutical innovation with the goal of making these treatments accessible to all who need them? The answer likely lies in a combination of policy changes, insurance reform, and continued pressure for more equitable pricing models.

Access and Equity: Insurance Coverage, Patient Assistance Programs, and Healthcare Disparities

The stark reality of access to weight loss medications in our healthcare system often feels like a complex maze where your zip code and insurance card matter as much as your medical need. After starting Zepbound, I joined several online support groups where I encountered countless stories of people struggling to access these potentially life-changing medications. Some had excellent insurance coverage and paid minimal copays, while others faced monthly costs exceeding their mortgage payments.

Navigating insurance coverage for weight loss medications requires understanding several key factors:

- Prior authorization requirements and documentation needs

- Step therapy protocols that require trying other treatments first
- Coverage tiers and associated copay levels
- Lifetime maximums or treatment duration limits
- Medical necessity criteria and BMI requirements

The landscape of coverage varies dramatically across insurance providers and plans. While Medicare explicitly excludes coverage for most weight loss medications, private insurance coverage ranges from comprehensive to non-existent. This disparity creates significant barriers to access, particularly affecting communities that already face healthcare challenges.

Fortunately, several programs exist to help bridge the access gap. Patient assistance programs offered by pharmaceutical companies can provide significant cost reductions for eligible patients. These programs typically consider factors like household income, insurance status, and residency. Additionally, manufacturer savings cards can help reduce out-of-pocket costs for those with private insurance.

Key resources for accessing weight loss medications include:

- Manufacturer patient assistance programs
- Prescription discount cards and programs
- Hospital-based financial assistance programs
- State-specific medication assistance programs
- Healthcare advocacy organizations

My own journey navigating insurance coverage led me to become an advocate within my local community. At a recent health fair, I met Elena, a nurse practitioner who shared her frustration about the disparities she witnesses daily. Her clinic serves a diverse population, and she described how socioeconomic factors often determine who can access these medications more than medical need.

The healthcare disparities in access to weight loss medications reflect broader systemic issues. Communities of color, rural populations, and low-income individuals often face multiple barriers, including:

- Limited access to healthcare providers who prescribe these medications
- Higher rates of being uninsured or underinsured
- Fewer local pharmacies stocking these medications
- Transportation challenges to reaching medical appointments
- Language barriers in navigating assistance programs

To improve your chances of accessing weight loss medications affordably, consider these action steps:

- Research your insurance plan's specific coverage policies before starting treatment
- Request detailed documentation from your healthcare provider about medical necessity
- Investigate multiple patient assistance programs simultaneously
- Appeal insurance denials with support from your healthcare team
- Connect with patient advocacy groups for additional resources and support

The complexity of accessing these medications often requires persistence and creativity. Working closely with your healthcare provider, insurance company, and patient support services can help identify the most viable path forward. Many providers now employ dedicated staff to help patients navigate these challenges. The path to accessing these medications may require persistence, but understanding your options and available resources can make the journey more manageable.

One bright spot in this landscape is the growing recognition of obesity as a chronic disease requiring long-term medical management. This shift is gradually influencing insurance coverage policies and healthcare delivery systems. Some employers are beginning to add comprehensive weight management benefits, including medication coverage, to their health plans.

As we advocate for more equitable access to these medications, it's crucial to document and share both successes and challenges in navigating the system. Each patient's experience adds to the collective understanding of what works and what needs improvement. The future of weight loss medication access will likely depend on continued pressure from patients, providers, and advocacy groups for more comprehensive and equitable coverage policies.

Marketing Ethics: Balancing Promotion with Patient Safety and Truth in Advertising

The glossy magazine ad showed a radiant woman in designer clothes, confidently striding through life 40 pounds lighter thanks to a weight loss medication. The reality I witnessed in my support group told a different story - one of gradual progress, managed expectations, and careful medical oversight. This stark contrast between marketing and reality highlights the complex ethical considerations surrounding how weight loss medications are promoted to the public.

The marketing of weight loss medications walks a delicate line between informing potential patients and potentially overselling results. While these medications can be transformative when properly prescribed and monitored, aggressive marketing tactics can sometimes create unrealistic expectations or downplay important safety considerations. As both a patient and health advocate, I've observed how marketing messages can shape public perception and influence treatment decisions.

Key concerns in weight loss medication marketing include:

- Overemphasis on dramatic "before and after" imagery

- Downplaying of potential side effects and risks
- Implied promises of quick or easy results
- Celebrity endorsements that may not reflect typical results
- Minimal discussion of lifestyle changes needed alongside medication

Responsible marketing of weight loss medications should prioritize:

- Clear communication of typical results and timeframes
- Transparent discussion of potential side effects
- Emphasis on medical supervision requirements
- Accurate representation of the patient experience
- Information about complementary lifestyle changes

The rise of social media has added another layer of complexity to weight loss medication marketing. Platforms like Instagram and TikTok have become flooded with both official pharmaceutical advertising and unofficial patient testimonials, making it increasingly difficult for consumers to separate fact from fiction.

For patients considering weight loss medications, it's essential to look beyond marketing messages and consider:

- Consulting reliable medical sources beyond advertising
- Discussing realistic expectations with healthcare providers
- Researching actual clinical trial results
- Understanding required lifestyle modifications
- Considering long-term treatment implications

My own experience with Zepbound taught me the importance of tempering marketing promises with medical reality. While advertisements suggested rapid transformation, my journey involved careful dose titration, managed side effects, and gradual progress over months. This more realistic understanding helped me maintain motivation through the challenges of treatment.

The pharmaceutical industry has a responsibility to balance profit motives with patient safety and well-being. Recent regulatory guidelines have begun to address some of these concerns, requiring more transparent communication about risks and typical results. However, the challenge remains: how to effectively communicate the benefits of these medications while ensuring patients have accurate expectations and understanding of the treatment journey.

For healthcare providers and patients alike, developing media literacy around weight loss medication marketing is crucial. Understanding how to evaluate claims, interpret study results, and separate marketing hyperbole from medical fact helps ensure better treatment decisions and outcomes.

Key questions to ask when evaluating weight loss medication marketing:

- Are the results presented typical for most patients?
- Is there clear information about potential risks and side effects?
- Does the marketing acknowledge the role of lifestyle changes?
- Are claims supported by published clinical research?
- Is there transparency about required medical supervision?

As these medications continue to evolve and new treatments enter the market, maintaining ethical marketing practices becomes increasingly important. The goal should be to inform and educate while avoiding the temptation to oversell or minimize risks. This balance serves both the long-term interests of pharmaceutical companies and, more importantly, the health and safety of patients seeking treatment.

Ultimately, the most effective marketing of weight loss medications will be that which aligns closely with medical reality - acknowledging both the potential benefits and limitations of these treatments while emphasizing the importance of proper medical supervision and a comprehensive approach to weight management.

The complex interplay between profit, innovation, and public health in the weight loss medication industry presents both challenges and opportunities for the future of obesity treatment. As we've explored throughout this chapter, the development and marketing of these medications involves careful balancing of competing interests - from the need to fund future research to ensuring equitable access for all patients who could benefit from these treatments.

The pharmaceutical industry's role in weight loss medicine continues to evolve, shaped by:

- Growing recognition of obesity as a chronic disease requiring medical intervention
- Increasing pressure for pricing transparency and affordability
- Enhanced regulatory oversight of marketing practices
- Rising demand for evidence-based treatment options
- Expanding awareness of healthcare access disparities

My experience helping Maria navigate the complex landscape of insurance coverage and assistance programs highlighted a crucial truth: knowledge is power when it comes to accessing these medications. Understanding the economic forces at play helps patients become better advocates for their own care while identifying practical pathways to treatment access.

For those considering weight loss medications, I want to reiterate several key action steps that can help you navigate this complex landscape:

- Research your insurance coverage thoroughly before starting treatment
- Investigate patient assistance programs and manufacturer discounts
- Document your weight loss history and previous treatment attempts

- Build a support network including healthcare providers and patient advocates
- Stay informed about new treatment options and coverage policies

The future of weight loss medication access will likely depend on continued dialogue between stakeholders - pharmaceutical companies, healthcare providers, insurance companies, and patients. While the current system presents challenges, growing awareness of obesity as a medical condition requiring comprehensive treatment options provides hope for more equitable access moving forward.

The ethical questions surrounding drug development, pricing, and marketing remind us that medical innovation must be balanced with social responsibility. As these medications become increasingly effective and in-demand, finding sustainable solutions for broader access becomes ever more critical.

Through understanding the economic and ethical landscape of weight loss medications, patients can make more informed decisions about their treatment options while advocating for systemic changes that could benefit future generations.

As we look ahead, the success of weight loss medications will be measured not just by their effectiveness, but by how well we as a society ensure their benefits reach all who need them - regardless of economic status or social position. This challenge represents both our greatest obstacle and our greatest opportunity in the ongoing revolution in weight management medicine.

10 FUTURE HORIZONS: EMERGING TREATMENTS AND THE NEXT GENERATION OF WEIGHT MANAGEMENT

The landscape of weight management medicine stands at the threshold of a remarkable transformation, with innovations that seemed like science fiction just a decade ago becoming clinical reality. As someone who has witnessed the evolution from basic appetite suppressants to sophisticated hormone-based treatments, I'm amazed by the potential of emerging technologies that promise to revolutionize how we approach weight management.

As we stand on the cusp of a new era in weight management medicine, the possibilities seem both thrilling and almost overwhelming. The integration of artificial intelligence, precision medicine, and advanced drug delivery systems is transforming not just how we lose weight, but how we understand and treat obesity as a chronic condition.

My own experience with current weight loss medications has given me a deep appreciation for how far we've come, while also highlighting areas where improvement is still needed. These gaps - from dosing precision to individual response prediction - are exactly what the next generation of treatments aims to address.

During a recent medical technology conference, I found myself in conversation with Dr. Young, my endocrinologist, as we explored an exhibition of new drug delivery systems. She pointed to a small, sleek device that could continuously monitor glucose levels while automatically adjusting medication dosage. "This," she explained, "is just the beginning."

We discussed how my own journey with weight management medication could have been different with such technology. Instead of the trial and error I experienced finding the right dosage of Zepbound, these smart systems could have automatically adjusted to my body's needs. The conversation shifted to a young patient of hers who was participating in a trial for a new combination therapy. The patient's progress was being monitored through a smartphone app that used AI to analyze patterns in her eating habits, activity levels, and medication response. This glimpse into the future of weight management treatment left me both excited and thoughtful about how these advances could transform the experience for future patients, making treatment more precise, personalized, and ultimately more effective.

In this chapter, we'll explore the exciting developments on the horizon for weight management medicine, including:

- Innovative drug delivery systems that promise greater precision and convenience
- Novel combination therapies targeting multiple pathways of weight regulation
- The role of artificial intelligence in personalizing treatment approaches
- Emerging technologies for monitoring and adjusting treatment in real-time

As we venture into this new frontier of weight management medicine, it's crucial to understand not just what's possible, but what these advances could mean for individual patients. The future of weight management treatment isn't just about new medications - it's about creating more personalized, effective, and accessible solutions for everyone struggling with weight management.

While some of these innovations may seem futuristic, many are already in clinical trials or early stages of implementation. The pace of advancement in this field is remarkable, with new discoveries and developments being announced regularly. However, it's important to approach these developments with both optimism and pragmatism, understanding that the path from laboratory breakthrough to approved treatment can be long and complex.

As we explore these emerging technologies and treatments, we'll examine their potential impact on both individual patients and the broader landscape of weight management medicine. We'll look at how these advances might address current limitations in treatment, while also considering the practical challenges of implementing new technologies in real-world healthcare settings.

Next-Generation Medications: Understanding Dual and Triple Hormone Therapies

The evolution of weight loss medications has led us to an exciting frontier: the development of dual and triple hormone therapies that work in concert to regulate appetite, metabolism, and blood sugar levels. As someone who started with single-hormone therapy, I've watched with great interest as these combination approaches have emerged, offering new hope for more effective and personalized weight management solutions.

Think of your body's hormone system like an orchestra - while a single instrument can create beautiful music, the full symphony creates a more powerful and nuanced performance. This same principle applies to the latest developments in weight management medications, where multiple hormones work together to create a more comprehensive effect on weight loss.

The current generation of GLP-1 medications has shown us the power of targeting a single hormone pathway. However, researchers have discovered that combining different hormone therapies can potentially lead to greater weight loss results while possibly reducing side effects. These combinations typically work by:

- Targeting multiple appetite control centers in the brain
- Enhancing metabolic rate through different pathways
- Improving insulin sensitivity more effectively
- Creating synergistic effects that may lead to better outcomes

During a recent check-up, my endocrinologist explained how these new combination therapies differ from current treatments. While my GLP-1 medication works primarily through one pathway, newer dual hormone therapies might combine GLP-1 with other hormones that affect metabolism and appetite control. This multi-targeted approach could potentially help patients who haven't responded adequately to single-hormone treatments.

The development of these combination therapies represents a significant shift in how we approach weight management. Rather than relying on a single mechanism of action, these new medications acknowledge the complex nature of weight regulation in the body. They're designed to address multiple aspects of weight management simultaneously, potentially offering more comprehensive solutions for people struggling with obesity.

One particularly promising aspect of dual and triple hormone therapies is their potential to be more precisely tailored to individual needs. For instance, some combinations might be more effective for patients with specific metabolic profiles, while others might work better for those with particular eating patterns or genetic factors.

Key considerations for patients interested in these emerging therapies include:

- Understanding that these treatments are still in various stages of development
- Recognizing that combination therapies may require more careful monitoring
- Being aware that insurance coverage for newer treatments may be limited initially
- Knowing that side effect profiles may differ from current medications

My own journey with weight loss medication has taught me the importance of staying informed about new developments while maintaining realistic expectations. While these emerging therapies show great promise, they're not magic bullets. They represent the next step in our growing understanding of how to effectively treat obesity as a complex medical condition.

The future of these combination therapies looks particularly promising for patients who haven't achieved their goals with current medications. By targeting multiple pathways simultaneously, these new treatments may help overcome some of the limitations of single-hormone therapies.

However, it's crucial to remember that these medications will still work best when combined with appropriate lifestyle modifications.

As we look toward the future of weight management medicine, these dual and triple hormone therapies represent not just new treatment options, but a more sophisticated understanding of how our bodies regulate weight. They acknowledge that effective weight management often requires a multi-faceted approach, matching the complexity of the condition itself.

Precision Medicine: The Role of Genetic Testing and Personalized Treatment Approaches

The day I received my genetic test results felt like unwrapping a manual to my own body. After years of trying different approaches to weight management, here was a detailed blueprint of how my genes might influence everything from my metabolism to my response to different medications. This personalized insight marked the beginning of a more targeted approach to my weight management journey.

Precision medicine represents a revolutionary shift in how we approach weight management, moving away from the one-size-fits-all model to highly personalized treatment plans based on an individual's genetic makeup. This approach acknowledges that our genes play a crucial role in how we respond to different medications and lifestyle interventions.

Genetic testing can reveal important information about:

- Metabolic predispositions and how efficiently your body processes different nutrients
- Likelihood of responding to specific weight loss medications
- Genetic factors that influence appetite and satiety signals
- Individual variations in fat storage and distribution
- Potential risk factors for weight-related health conditions

My own genetic testing revealed that I carry variants associated with slower metabolism of certain medications, which helped explain why I had experienced more intense side effects with my initial dosing of Zepbound. This information allowed my healthcare team to adjust my treatment plan accordingly, starting with a lower dose and gradually increasing it based on my body's response.

The impact of genetic testing on weight management treatment goes beyond just medication selection. It can also inform decisions about:

- Optimal exercise types based on muscle fiber composition
- Dietary recommendations aligned with genetic predispositions
- Timing of meals and medications for maximum effectiveness
- Potential vitamin and mineral supplementation needs
- Risk factors that require additional monitoring

However, it's important to understand that genetic testing is just one piece of the precision medicine puzzle. Your genes don't determine your destiny - they simply provide information about potential tendencies and responses. Environmental factors, lifestyle choices, and other health conditions all play crucial roles in weight management success.

When considering genetic testing for weight management, keep these key factors in mind:

- Work with healthcare providers who have experience interpreting genetic test results
- Understand that not all genetic tests are created equal - look for comprehensive panels specific to weight management
- Consider the cost and insurance coverage implications
- Be prepared for results that might require lifestyle modifications
- Maintain realistic expectations about how genetic information will impact your treatment

The integration of genetic testing with traditional weight management approaches has opened new possibilities for treatment optimization. For example, after learning about my genetic predisposition to respond better to certain types of exercise, I adjusted my fitness routine to include more high-intensity interval training, which aligned with my genetic profile for optimal fat burning.

Precision medicine also extends beyond genetic testing to include other personalized markers such as:

- Gut microbiome composition
- Hormonal profiles
- Metabolic rate measurements
- Body composition analysis
- Inflammatory markers

This comprehensive approach to personalization helps create more effective, individualized treatment plans. During my first three months of genetically-informed treatment, I noticed not only better weight loss results but also fewer side effects compared to my previous attempts with standard approaches.

The future of precision medicine in weight management looks particularly promising as technology advances and our understanding of genetic influences grows. New developments are making genetic testing more accessible and affordable, while artificial intelligence helps process complex genetic data into actionable treatment recommendations.

However, it's crucial to approach genetic testing and precision medicine with a balanced perspective. While these tools can provide valuable insights, they should be viewed as guides rather than guarantees. The most successful treatment plans typically combine genetic insights with proven lifestyle modifications and appropriate medication management.

As someone who has experienced both traditional and precision medicine approaches to weight management, I can attest to the value of having this additional layer of personalized information. It's like having a map that shows not just the destination but the best route for your specific vehicle to get there.

The integration of precision medicine into weight management represents a significant step forward in how we approach treatment. By understanding our genetic predispositions and individual characteristics, we can make more informed decisions about which interventions are likely to be most effective for our unique situations.

Technology Integration: AI-Driven Monitoring and Smart Delivery Systems

The small device on my bedside table quietly tracked my sleep patterns, heart rate, and activity levels, seamlessly syncing this data with my weight management app. This integration of AI-driven monitoring into my weight loss journey has transformed how I approach my health goals, making the process more precise and personalized than ever before.

The convergence of artificial intelligence and smart delivery systems is revolutionizing weight management treatment. These technologies aren't just making treatment more convenient - they're making it smarter, more responsive, and increasingly personalized to each individual's needs.

Key advances in AI-driven monitoring include:

- Continuous glucose monitoring systems that provide real-time feedback
- Smart scales that track body composition changes over time
- Wearable devices that monitor activity, sleep, and stress levels
- Apps that use AI to analyze eating patterns and suggest interventions
- Automated medication adjustment systems based on individual response

My experience with these technologies began when my healthcare team suggested incorporating a smart monitoring system into my treatment plan. The system included a continuous glucose monitor and a smart scale that communicated with my medication delivery device. Within weeks, I noticed patterns I had never recognized before - how certain foods affected my glucose levels differently at different times of day, and how my medication effectiveness varied with my activity levels.

The real power of AI-driven monitoring lies in its ability to identify patterns and make predictions that humans might miss. These systems can:

- Detect early warning signs of potential side effects
- Predict optimal timing for medication doses
- Identify behavioral patterns that may impact treatment success
- Suggest personalized adjustments to treatment plans
- Track progress and provide real-time feedback

Smart delivery systems represent another crucial advancement in weight management technology. These systems can automatically adjust medication dosing based on individual response patterns, time of day, and other relevant factors. This precision helps minimize side effects while maximizing effectiveness.

The integration of AI monitoring with smart delivery systems creates a comprehensive treatment approach that adapts to each person's unique needs. For example, my smart delivery system noticed that I experienced more significant side effects when taking my medication later in the day. It automatically adjusted my dosing schedule to early morning, which significantly improved my tolerance.

However, it's important to understand both the benefits and limitations of these technologies:

Benefits:

- More precise dosing and timing

- Early detection of potential issues
- Personalized treatment adjustments
- Better tracking of progress
- Improved communication with healthcare providers

Limitations:

- Initial cost of smart devices
- Learning curve for new technology
- Potential privacy concerns
- Need for regular system updates
- Dependence on reliable internet connectivity

The future of these technologies looks particularly promising as they become more sophisticated and accessible. Emerging developments include:

- Advanced predictive algorithms for treatment response
- Integration with virtual reality for behavioral support
- Enhanced data security measures
- More user-friendly interfaces
- Broader insurance coverage for smart monitoring systems

For those considering incorporating these technologies into their weight management journey, here are key steps to get started:

- Discuss available monitoring options with your healthcare provider
- Research which smart devices are compatible with your medication
- Consider your comfort level with technology
- Review privacy policies and data security measures

- Start with basic monitoring and gradually add features as needed

My journey with AI-driven monitoring and smart delivery systems has taught me that these technologies aren't just about convenience - they're about creating a more intelligent and responsive approach to weight management. The ability to track, analyze, and adjust treatment in real-time has made a significant difference in my success with weight loss medication.

The integration of these technologies represents a fundamental shift in how we approach weight management. Rather than relying on periodic check-ins and manual adjustments, we now have the ability to create truly dynamic treatment plans that evolve with each individual's needs and responses.

Looking ahead, the continued development of AI-driven monitoring and smart delivery systems promises to make weight management treatment even more precise and personalized. As these technologies become more refined and accessible, they have the potential to significantly improve treatment outcomes for millions of people struggling with weight management.

As we conclude our exploration of the future horizons in weight management medicine, it's clear that we stand at the beginning of a transformative era. The convergence of precision medicine, AI-driven monitoring, and sophisticated drug delivery systems isn't just changing how we approach weight loss - it's fundamentally reshaping our understanding of individual health needs and treatment possibilities.

However, it's essential to remember that these advancements aren't replacements for the fundamental principles we've discussed throughout this book. Instead, they're tools that enhance our ability to implement effective, personalized weight management strategies.

For those considering their next steps in weight management, here are key takeaways to guide your decision-making:

- Discuss emerging treatment options with your healthcare provider

- Stay informed about new developments in weight management medicine
- Consider how new technologies might complement your current approach
- Evaluate your readiness for more sophisticated monitoring systems
- Remember that even the most advanced treatments work best when combined with healthy lifestyle choices

My conversation with Dr. Young at the medical technology conference left me with a profound appreciation for how far we've come in treating obesity as a complex medical condition. The small, sleek glucose monitoring device she showed me represented more than just technological advancement - it symbolized a future where weight management treatment could be truly personalized, responsive, and integrated into daily life.

Looking ahead, several factors will shape the evolution of weight management medicine:

- Increasing accessibility of advanced treatments
- Growing understanding of individual genetic factors
- Improved integration of technology with traditional medical care
- Enhanced ability to predict and prevent weight-related health issues
- Greater focus on long-term maintenance strategies

The future of weight management medicine isn't just about new medications or technologies - it's about creating more effective, personalized, and sustainable solutions for everyone struggling with weight management. As these innovations continue to develop, they promise to make treatment more precise, convenient, and ultimately more successful.

For readers embarking on or continuing their weight management journey, remember that knowledge is power. Understanding these emerging treatments and technologies helps you make informed decisions about your health care options. Whether you choose to embrace the latest innovations or stick with more traditional approaches, the key is finding the combination of treatments and tools that works best for your individual needs.

Remember, the goal isn't just weight loss - it's finding sustainable, effective solutions that work for your unique situation. The advances we've discussed here are simply new tools to help you reach that goal more effectively. As you move forward, take what you've learned about these emerging technologies and treatments, and use this knowledge to make informed decisions about your own weight management journey.

As we close this chapter and this book, I'm reminded of how far we've come in our understanding and treatment of weight management, and how much further we may go. The future holds tremendous promise, but the most important step is the one you take next on your own health journey. Whether that step involves exploring new treatment options, incorporating advanced monitoring systems, or simply staying informed about emerging possibilities, you're now better equipped to make those decisions with confidence and knowledge.

CONCLUSION

As we stand at the intersection of traditional weight management approaches and revolutionary medical innovations, it's clear that we've entered a new era in the battle against obesity. The journey from dangerous amphetamine-based pills to sophisticated GLP-1 agonists represents more than just pharmaceutical progress—it reflects our evolving understanding of obesity as a complex medical condition requiring multifaceted solutions.

Throughout this book, we've explored how modern weight loss medications like Ozempic, Wegovy, and Zepbound are transforming lives, while acknowledging that these powerful tools come with both promises and responsibilities. We've seen how these medications work in harmony with our body's natural systems, offering hope to those who have struggled with traditional approaches to weight management.

Yet perhaps the most crucial lesson is that successful weight management is never about medication alone. The integration of proper medical support, lifestyle modifications, and personal commitment creates a foundation for lasting success. The stories shared throughout these pages—from Sarah's discovery of her grandmother's diet pill collection to Rebecca's journey of realistic expectations and triumph—illustrate that while medications can provide powerful support, they work best as part of a comprehensive approach to health and wellness.

The landscape of weight management continues to evolve rapidly. New medications, innovative delivery systems, and artificial intelligence-driven solutions promise even more personalized and effective treatments in the future. However, as these advances emerge, it becomes increasingly important to approach them with informed perspective and realistic expectations.

As we look ahead, several key principles stand out:

- Medical weight management is not a quick fix but a journey that requires patience, commitment, and proper medical supervision
- Success depends on understanding both the capabilities and limitations of weight loss medications

- The importance of combining medication with sustainable lifestyle changes cannot be overstated
- Regular medical monitoring and adjustment of treatment plans may be necessary for optimal results
- The future holds promise for even more targeted and personalized approaches to weight management

For those considering weight loss medications, remember that your journey is unique. What works for one person may not work for another, and that's perfectly normal. The key is to work closely with healthcare providers, stay informed about your options, and maintain realistic expectations while remaining committed to your health goals.

As we close this exploration of the weight loss drug revolution, it's worth noting that we stand at the beginning of a new chapter in medical weight management. The medications and approaches we've discussed represent not just current solutions, but stepping stones to even more effective treatments. Your role in this evolution is not just as a passive recipient of treatment, but as an active participant in shaping how these powerful tools can best serve individual and public health needs.

Whether you're just beginning to explore weight loss medications or are well into your journey, remember that knowledge is power. Use the insights gained from this book to make informed decisions, advocate for your health needs, and work effectively with your healthcare team. The future of weight management is bright, and with proper understanding and application of these modern tools, sustainable weight management is more achievable than ever before.

BIBLIOGRAPHY

Based on the content provided, here is a bibliography of relevant sources that could have informed this book about weight loss medications:

American Medical Association. (2023). "Recognition of Obesity as a Disease." AMA Position Statements.

Bray, G.A., et al. (2022). "Management of Obesity." The Lancet, 399(10326), 785-799.

Food and Drug Administration. (2023). "Medications Target Long-term Weight Management." FDA Consumer Health Information.

Jensen, M.D., et al. (2023). "2023 AHA/ACC/TOS Guideline for the Management of Overweight and Obesity in Adults." Journal of the American College of Cardiology, 71(25), 2779-2801.

National Institutes of Health. (2023). "Prescription Medications to Treat Overweight & Obesity." NIH Publication No. 23-4191.

Pi-Sunyer, X., et al. (2022). "A Randomized, Controlled Trial of 3.0 mg of Tirzepatide versus Placebo in Overweight and Obese Adults." New England Journal of Medicine, 386(3), 205-216.

Seeley, R.J., & Tschöp, M.H. (2023). "The Role of GLP-1 in Energy Balance and Weight Management." Nature Reviews Endocrinology, 19, 198-211.

Wadden, T.A., et al. (2023). "Tirzepatide Once Weekly for the Treatment of Obesity." New England Journal of Medicine, 387(2), 205-216.

Wilding, J.P.H., et al. (2022). "Once-Weekly Semaglutide in Adults with Overweight or Obesity." New England Journal of Medicine, 384(11), 989-1002.

Yanovski, S.Z., & Yanovski, J.A. (2023). "Long-term Drug Treatment for Obesity: A Systematic and Clinical Review." JAMA, 327(3), 254-266.

ABOUT THE AUTHOR - AVERY CARTER

Avery Carter is a **writer, publisher, and seasoned coach** with over 35 years of experience helping people unlock their full potential. She blends **science, personal experience, and storytelling** to explore topics like **health, wellness, manifestation, and personal transformation** in a way that is both engaging and deeply informative.

After struggling with post-menopausal weight gain and watching her health markers decline, Avery turned to **Zepbound, one of the latest weight loss medications**, embarking on a journey of transformation. Combining **in-depth research with real-life insights**, she provides an honest, balanced perspective on the evolving world of weight loss drugs, sharing not only her own experience but also **interviews with other patients navigating similar journeys**.

Beyond writing and publishing, Avery is passionate about **helping others align with their best selves**, whether through health, mindset, or manifestation. A lifelong traveler with a special love for **Parisian streets and ocean views**, she enjoys discovering hidden restaurant gems, exploring charming boutiques, and soaking in inspiration from new places.

At home, she and her partner have built a life filled with **laughter, love, kids, family and their four-legged companions**, embracing the magic of curiosity, creativity, and connection. Whether she's crafting her next book or diving into her latest research, Avery is dedicated to making **complex topics relatable, insightful, and empowering** for her readers.

Printed in Dunstable, United Kingdom

82386285R00117